Study Guide for

Nursing Research: Methods and Critical Appraisal for Evidence-Based Practice

Ninth Edition

Geri LoBiondo-Wood, PhD, RN, FAAN
Professor and Coordinator, PhD in Nursing Program
University of Texas Health Science Center at Houston
School of Nursing
Houston, Texas

Judith Haber, PhD, RN, FAAN
The Ursula Springer Leadership Professor in Nursing
New York University
Rory Meyers College of Nursing
New York, New York

Study Guide prepared by:

Carey A. Berry, MS, BSN, RN
Formerly, Clinical Nurse
Gastrointestinal Surgical Oncology
M.D. Anderson Cancer Center
The University of Texas
Houston, Texas

ELSEVIER

ELSEVIER

3251 Riverport Lane
St. Louis, Missouri 63043

STUDY GUIDE FOR NURSING RESEARCH: METHODS AND CRITICAL APPRAISAL FOR EVIDENCE-BASED PRACTICE, NINTH EDITION

ISBN: 978-0-323-44761-4

Notices

Knowledge and best practice in this field are constantly changing. As new research and experience broaden our understanding, changes in research methods, professional practices, or medical treatment may become necessary.

Practitioners and researchers must always rely on their own experience and knowledge in evaluating and using any information, methods, compounds, or experiments described herein. In using such information or methods, they should be mindful of their own safety and the safety of others, including parties for whom they have a professional responsibility.

With respect to any drug or pharmaceutical products identified, readers are advised to check the most current information provided (i) on procedures featured or (ii) by the manufacturer of each product to be administered and to verify the recommended dose or formula, the method and duration of administration, and contraindications. It is the responsibility of practitioners, relying on their own experience and knowledge of their patients, to make diagnoses, to determine dosages and the best treatment for each individual patient, and to take all appropriate safety precautions.

To the fullest extent of the law, neither the Publisher nor the authors, contributors, or editors assume any liability for any injury and/or damage to persons or property as a matter of products liability, negligence or otherwise, or from any use or operation of any methods, products, instructions, or ideas contained in the material herein.

Executive Content Strategist: Lee Henderson
Content Development Manager: Lisa Newton
Content Development Specialist: Melissa Rawe
Publishing Services Manager: Deepthi Unni
Project Manager: Nadhiya Sekar
Design Direction: Muthukumaran Thangaraj

Printed in the United States of America

Last digit is the print number: 9 8 7 6 5 4 3 2 1

Introduction

Information bombards us! The student lament used to be, "I can't find any information on X." Now the cry is, "What do I do with all of the information on X?" The focus shifts from finding information to thinking about how to use and filter information. What information is worth keeping? What should be discarded? What is useful to clinical practice? What is fluff? Where are the gaps?

Thinking about the links between information and practice is critical to the improvement of the nursing care we deliver. As each of us strengthens our individual understanding of the links between interventions and outcomes, we move nursing's collective practice closer to being truly evidence based. We can "know" what intervention works best in what situation.

"Helping people get better safely and efficiently" begins with thinking. Our intent is that the activities in the Study Guide will help you strengthen your skills in thinking about information found in the literature. The activities are designed to assist you in evaluating the research you read so you are prepared to undertake the critical analysis of research studies. As you practice the appraisal skills addressed in this Study Guide, you will be strengthening your ability to make evidence-based practice decisions grounded in theory and research.

What an incredible time to be a nurse!

GENERAL DIRECTIONS

1. We recommend that you read the textbook chapter first, then complete the Study Guide activities for that chapter.

2. Complete each Study Guide chapter in order. The Study Guide is designed so that you build on the knowledge gained in Chapter 1 to complete the activities in Chapter 2, and so forth. The activities are designed to give you the opportunity to apply the knowledge learned in the textbook and actually use this knowledge to solve problems, thereby gaining increased confidence that comes only from working through each chapter.

3. Follow the specific directions that precede each activity. Be certain that you have the resources needed to complete the activity before you begin.

4. Take the posttest in each Study Guide chapter after you have completed all of the chapter's activities. The answers for the posttest items can be found in the answer key. If you answer 85% of the questions correctly, be confident that you have grasped the essential material presented in the chapter.

5. Clarify any questions, confusion, or concerns you may have with your instructor.

ACTIVITY ANSWERS ARE IN THE BACK OF THIS BOOK

Answers in a workbook such as this do not follow a formula like answers in a math book. Many times you are asked to make a judgment about a particular problem. If your judgment differs from that of the authors, review the criteria that you used to make your decision. Determine if you followed a logical progression of steps to reach your conclusion. If not, rework the activity. If the process you followed appears logical, and your answer remains different, remember that even experts may disagree on many of the judgment calls in nursing research. There will continue to be many "gray areas." If you average an 85% agreement with the authors, you can be sure that you are on the right track and should feel very confident about your level of expertise.

Carey A. Berry, MS, BSN, RN

Contents

1 Integrating Research, Evidence-Based Practice, and Quality Improvement Processes

INTRODUCTION

One goal of this chapter is to assist you in reviewing the material presented in Chapter 1 of the text written by LoBiondo-Wood and Haber. A second and more fundamental goal is to provide you with an opportunity to begin practicing the role of a critical consumer of research. Succeeding chapters in this study guide fine-tune your ability to evaluate research studies critically.

LEARNING OUTCOMES

On completion of this chapter, you should be able to do the following:

- State the significance of research to evidence-based nursing practice and quality improvement.
- Identify the role of the consumer of nursing research.
- Define *evidence-based practice.*
- Define *quality improvement.*
- Discuss evidence-based and quality improvement decision making.
- Explain the difference between quantitative and qualitative research.
- Explain the difference among types of systematic reviews.
- Identify the importance of critical reading skills for critical appraisal of research studies.
- Discuss the format and style of research reports and articles.
- Discuss how to use an evidence hierarchy when critically appraising research studies.

Activity 1

Match the term in Column B with the appropriate phrase in Column A. Each term will be used only once. This may be a good time to review the glossary and the key terms in Chapter 1.

Column A

1. ________ Systematic investigation about phenomena
2. ________ Studies conducted to understand the meaning of human experience
3. ________ Statistical technique used to summarize studies in a systematic review
4. ________ Critically evaluates a research report's content based on a set of criteria to evaluate the scientific merit for application to practice
5. ________ Studies conducted to test relationships, assess differences, and/or explain cause and effect
6. ________ Summary and assessment of a group that considered similar research questions
7. ________ Clinical practice based on the collection, evaluation, and integration of clinical expertise, research evidence, and patient preferences
8. ________ Systematically developed statements that provide recommendations to guide practice
9. ________ Systematic use of data to monitor outcomes of care
10. ________ Brief summary of a study found at the beginning of an article
11. ________ Review and synthesis that may include qualitative and quantitative articles in a focused area
12. ________ Guidelines developed using published research findings
13. ________ Synthesis of qualitative research studies on a focused topic using specific qualitative methodology
14. ________ Expert-based guidelines, developed by agreement of experts in a field
15. ________ Rating system or hierarchy for assessing the relative worth of qualitative and quantitative studies
16. ________ Skill in evaluating the appropriateness of the content of a research article, applying standards or critiquing criteria to assess the study's scientific merit for use in practice, or considering alternative ways of handling the same topic
17. ________ Evaluating the strengths and weaknesses of a research article for scientific merit and application to practice, theory, education, or needing more research

Column B

a. Critique
b. Meta-analysis
c. Research
d. Qualitative
e. Systematic review
f. Evidence-based practice
g. Quantitative
h. Clinical guidelines
i. Quality improvement
j. Abstract
k. Consensus guidelines
l. Critical appraisal
m. Critical reading
n. Evidence-based guidelines
o. Meta-synthesis
p. Levels of evidence
q. Integrative review

Activity 2

Match the term in Column B with the appropriate phrase in Column A. Terms from Column B will be used more than once.

Column A

1. _______ Getting a general sense of the material
2. _______ Clarifying unfamiliar terms with text
3. _______ Using constructive skepticism
4. _______ Questioning assumptions
5. _______ Rationally examining ideas
6. _______ Thinking about your own thinking
7. _______ Allowing assessment of study validity

Column B

a. Critical thinking

b. Critical reading

Activity 3

Complete each item with the appropriate word or phrase from the following list: parts, comprehensive, whole, preliminary

1. Key variables, new terms, and steps of the research process should be identified following a(n) _______________ understanding of a research article.
2. With _______________ understanding of a research article, you should be able to state the main purpose of the study in one or two sentences.
3. Analysis of an article will allow understanding of the _______________ of a study; synthesis will allow understanding of the _______________ article and all steps in the research process.

Activity 4: Evidence-Based Practice Activity

1. For Appendix B (Hawthorne et al., 2016), Appendix D (Turner-Sack et al., 2016), and Appendix E (Al-Mallah et al., 2016), identify the articles' level of evidence using Figure 1-1 in your textbook.
   a. Hawthorne et al., 2016: ____
   b. Turner-Sack et al., 2016: ____
   c. Al-Mallah et al., 2016: ____

Activity 5

Match the term in Column B with the appropriate phrase in Column A.

Column A

1. _______ Extent to which a study's design, implementation, and analysis minimize bias
2. _______ Degree to which studies that have similar and different designs, but consider the same research question, report similar findings
3. _______ Number of studies that have evaluated the research question, as well as the strength of the findings from the data analyses

Column B

a. Consistency
b. Quality
c. Quantity

Activity 6

Using Appendix A (Nyamathi et al., 2015), determine where in the article the following steps of the research process are identified:

1. Research problem: ______
2. Purpose: ______
3. Literature review: ______
4. Theoretical framework and/or conceptual framework: ______
5. Hypothesis/research questions: ______
6. Research design: ______
7. Sample—type and size: ______
8. Legal-ethical issues: ______
9. Instruments: ______
10. Validity and reliability: ______
11. Data collection procedure: ______
12. Data analysis: ______
13. Results: ______
14. Discussion of findings and new findings: ______
15. Implications, limitations, and recommendations: ______

POSTTEST

1. To read a research study critically, the reader must have skilled reading, writing, and reasoning abilities. Use these abilities to read the following abstract, and then identify concepts, clarify any unfamiliar concepts or terms, and question any assumptions or rationales presented.

   The purpose of this longitudinal study with a sample of Hispanic, Black non-Hispanic, and White non-Hispanic bereaved parents was to test the relationships between spiritual/religious coping strategies and grief, mental health (depression and post-traumatic stress disorder), and personal growth for mothers and fathers at 1 (T1) and 3 (T2) months after the infant's/child's death in the NICU/PICU, with and without control for race/ethnicity and religion... The sample for this study consisted of 165 bereaved parents (114 mothers/51 fathers) of 124 deceased infants/children (69 NICU and 55 PICU) recruited for the larger study from four level III NICUs and four tertiary care PICUs... Depression was measured with the Beck Depression Inventory (BDI-II) (Beck, Steer, & Brown, 1996). Parents rated each of the 21 items on a scale from 0 to 3 with higher summative scores indicating greater severity of depressive symptoms...Bereaved mothers' greater use of spiritual activities, but not religious activities, was significantly related to lower symptoms or grief (despair, detachment, and disorganization), depression and PTSD at T1 and T2... Bereaved fathers' greater use of spiritual activities was significantly related to lower symptoms of grief (despair, detachment, and disorganization) and depression at T1 and T2...Research studies have found that bereaved parents experience many emotional benefits associated with the use of religious coping to deal with their grief and mental health (Lichtenhal et al., 2010; Meert et al., 2005). In this study, religious activities were not effective in lowering symptoms of grief, depression, and PTSD for bereaved mothers at 1 month and fathers at 3 months post-death (Hawthorne et al., 2016).

   a. Identify the concepts.

   b. List any unfamiliar concepts or terms that you would need to clarify.

c. What assumptions or rationales would you question?

2. Identify one similarity between research and evidence-based practice.

3. Identify one difference between research and evidence-based practice.

4. Identify one similarity between quantitative and qualitative research.

5. Identify one difference between quantitative and qualitative research.

REFERENCES

Al-Malleh, M. H., Faraf, I., Al-Madani, W., Bdeir, B., AlHabib, S., Bigelow, M. L., . . . Ferwana, M. (2015). The impact of nurse-led clinics on mortality and morbidity of patients with cardiovascular diseases: A systematic review and meta-analysis. *Journal of Cardiovascular Nursing, 31*(1), 89-95.

Hawthorne, D. M., Youngblut, J. M., & Brooten, D. (2016). Parent spirituality, grief, and mental health at 1 year and 3 months after their infant's/child's death in an intensive care unit. *Journal of Pediatric Nursing, 31*, 73-80.

Nyamathi, A., Salem, B. E., Zhang, S., Farabee, D., Hall, B., Khalilifard, F., Leake, B. (2015). Nursing care management, peer coaching, and hepatitis A and B vaccine completion among homeless men recently released on parole. *Nursing Research, 64*(3), 177-189.

Turner-Sack, A. M., Menna, R., Setchell, S. R., Maan, C., & Cataudella, D. (2016). Psychological functioning, post traumatic growth, and coping in parents and siblings of adolescent cancer survivors. *Oncology Nursing Forum, 43*(1), 48-56.

2 Research Questions, Hypotheses, and Clinical Questions

INTRODUCTION

This chapter focuses on identifying research questions, hypotheses, and clinical questions. If developed correctly, research questions can be very helpful to you as a research consumer because they concisely describe the essence of the research study. Research questions present the idea that is to be examined in the study. Hypotheses, which extend from the literature review and research questions, are predictions that provide a vehicle for testing the relationships between variables. For the nurse who considers using the results of a given study in practice, the two primary concerns are to locate and critique the research question and the hypotheses. The research question or hypotheses provide the most succinct link between the underlying theoretical base and guide the design of the research study. Although similar to research questions, clinical questions are developed by the nurse to provide answers to clinical situations. Clinical questions, framed using the population, intervention, comparison, outcome (PICO) format, are the basis for searching the literature to identify the best available evidence for clinical situations.

LEARNING OUTCOMES

On completion of this chapter, you should be able to do the following:

- Describe how the research question and hypothesis relate to the other components of the research process.
- Describe the process of identifying and refining a research question or hypothesis.
- Discuss the appropriate use of research questions versus hypotheses in a research study.
- Identify the criteria for determining the significance of a research question or hypothesis.
- Discuss how the purpose, research question, and hypothesis suggest the level of evidence to be obtained from the findings of a research study.
- Discuss the purpose of developing a clinical question.
- Discuss the differences between a research question and a clinical question in relation to evidence-based practice.
- Apply critiquing criteria to the evaluation of a research question and hypothesis in a research report.

Activity 1

Match the terms in Column B to the appropriate phrase in Column A.

Column A

1. _______ Statement about the relationship among two or more variables
2. _______ Variable that has the presumed effect on another variable
3. _______ Nonmanipulated variable that the researcher is interested in understanding, explaining, or predicting
4. _______ Property of the research question that variables must lend themselves to observation, measurement, and analysis
5. _______ Concepts or properties that are operationalized and studied
6. _______ Statement that presents the idea(s) to be examined in the study

Column B

a. Testability
b. Independent variable
c. Variables
d. Dependent variable
e. Research question
f. Hypothesis

Activity 2

1. Read the following and choose the best description of the criteria used to determine significance of a research question response below:
   A. Knowledge derived from the study will potentially benefit patients, nurses, the medical community or society.
   B. Findings from the study could be used to support or show a lack of support for untested theoretical concepts.
   C. Findings will ensure further grant support for a new or existing research program.
   D. The results could support, fill gaps, or clarify conflicts within the literature.
   E. Nursing practices and/or policies may be developed, retained, or revised based on the findings.
   F. The results may influence nursing practice, education, or administration.
      a. All of the above
      b. A, B, C, D, E but not F
      c. None of the above
      d. A, B, D, E, F, but not C
      e. A, B, E, and F only

2. If a research question does not meet the criteria for significance, what is the next step?
   a. Revise the question extensively.
   b. Discard the question.
   c. Proceed with the study.
   d. Both A and B are correct.

Activity 3

The development of a research question or hypothesis is a key step that drives the research process. Identify when you would expect a research question, a hypothesis, or either a research question or hypothesis.

KEY:

a. Research question
b. Hypothesis
c. Research question or hypothesis

1. ________ May be explicitly stated or may be found buried in the purpose, aims, or goals or in the results section.
2. ________ Can be used to guide many types of research studies but is often used in exploratory, descriptive, qualitative, or hypothesis-generating studies.
3. ________ A declarative statement about the relationship between two or more variables that predicts the expected outcome of the study.
4. ________ Developed before the study is conducted and provides direction for data collection, analysis, and interpretation.
5. ________ Implies a relationship between variables; either causal or associative.
6. ________ Displays testability of variables by observation, measurement, and analysis.
7. ________ May anticipate the direction of the relationship between variables or may imply only a relationship between variables.
8. ________ May be answered by a quantitative or qualitative design.
9. ________ Includes a relationship statement, testability, and consistency with theory.
10. ________ Provides information about the intent of the study and suggests the level of evidence obtained by the findings.

Activity 4

A good research question exhibits three characteristics. Critique the following research questions to determine if each of the three criteria is present. Following each problem statement is a list representing the three criteria (A, B, and C). Circle *yes* or *no* to indicate whether each criterion is met.

The research question:

a. Clearly identifies the variable(s) under consideration
b. Specifies the population being studied
c. Implies the possibility of empirical testing

1. The purpose of this study was to first assess whether seronegative parolees previously randomized to any of three intervention conditions were more likely to complete the vaccine series as well as to identify the predictors of HAV/HBV vaccine completion (Nyamathi et al., 2015).
   Criterion A: Yes No
   Criterion B: Yes No
   Criterion C: Yes No

2. The purpose of this longitudinal study was to test the relationships between spiritual/religious coping strategies and grief, mental health (depression and post-traumatic stress disorder) and personal growth for mothers and fathers at 1 (T1) and 3 (T2) months after the infant's/child's death in the NICU/PICU with and without control for race/ethnicity and religion (Hawthorne et al., 2016).
   Criterion A: Yes No
   Criterion B: Yes No
   Criterion C: Yes No

3. To examine psychological functioning, post-traumatic growth (PTG), coping, and cancer-related characteristics of adolescent cancer survivors—parents and siblings (Turner-Sack et al., 2016).
   Criterion A: Yes No
   Criterion B: Yes No
   Criterion C: Yes No

Activity 5

The ability to distinguish between independent and dependent variables is crucial in critiquing a research hypothesis to determine whether it is a succinct statement of the relationship between two variables. In each of the following research hypotheses, determine (A) the independent variable and (B) the dependent variable and (C) label each as a DH (directional hypothesis) or NDH (nondirectional hypothesis).

1. Regular provision of iron improves iron status of breast-fed infants without adverse effects (Ziegler et al., 2009).
   a. Independent variable:

   b. Dependent variable:

   c.

2. There is no difference between continuous nebulization of albuterol at 7.5 mg/hr (usual dose) and 15 mg/hr (high dose) in peak flow improvement up to 3 hours in patients with acute bronchospasm (Stein & Levitt, 2003).
   a. Independent variable:

   b. Dependent variable:

   c.

3. People who report more frequent or more recent dental prophylaxes are more likely to have better glycemic control (Taylor et al., 2005).
   a. Independent variable:

   b. Dependent variable:

   c.

4. More supportive/less negative parenting is associated with lower resting blood pressure and heart rates in children (Bell & Belsky, 2008).
   a. Independent variable:

   b. Dependent variable:

   c.

Activity 6

Match the terms in column B to the appropriate phrase in column A. Terms may be used more than once.

Column A

1. _______ May be manipulated in experimental research studies
2. _______ Can relate to differences in another variable
3. _______ Is the variable the researcher is interested in understanding, explaining, or predicting
4. _______ May have more than one in a study
5. _______ Has the presumed effect on the dependent variable
6. _______ May be assumed to occur naturally before or during the study in non-experimental research
7. _______ Varies with a change in the independent variable
8. _______ Is not manipulated
9. _______ Takes on different values
10. _______ Symbolized by X
11. _______ Symbolized by Y

Column B

DV: dependent variable
IV: independent variable
Both: dependent variable and independent variable

Activity 7

Clinical questions often arise from clinical situations. Using the PICO format for formulating clinical questions helps practicing nurses identify the best available evidence on which to base clinical and health care decisions. In the following clinical questions, identify the four components of clinical questions.

1. In children presenting to the emergency department with acute long-bone fractures, is intranasal fentanyl equivalent to intravenous morphine for pain control? (Yost, 2007)

   P: ______________________________

   I: ______________________________

   C: ______________________________

   O: ______________________________

2. Is a group intervention for parents and children more effective than routine care for weight loss in obese school-age children? (Heale, 2008)

   P: ______________________________

   I: ______________________________

   C: ______________________________

   O: ______________________________

3. What are the experiences of men after laparoscopic radical prostatectomy? (Mick, 2009)

   P: ______________________________

   I: ______________________________

   C: ______________________________

   O: ______________________________

POSTTEST

Answer the following *true* (T) or *false* (F).

1. ________ Research questions are developed to provide answers to clinical situations.
2. ________ A hypothesis provides a prediction for testing relationships between variables.
3. ________ Variation in the dependent variable that is assumed to depend on changes in the independent variable implies causation.
4. ________ A hypothesis provides a prediction of the outcome of the study.
5. ________ Qualitative data are not useful as evidence in a research study.
6. ________ A hypothesis should be directional.
7. ________ The search for relevant literature and scientific evidence is guided by well-defined research questions.
8. ________ An independent variable in one study may act as a dependent or independent variable in another study.

REFERENCES

Bell, B. G., & Belsky, J. (2008). Parenting and children's cardiovascular functioning. *Child: Care, Health, and Development, 34*(2), 194-203.

Hawthorne, D. M., Youngblut, J. M., & Brooten, D. (2016). Patient spirituality, grief, and mental health at 1 and 3 months after their infant's/child's death in an intensive care unit. *Journal of Pediatric Nursing, 31*(1), 73-80.

Heale, R. (2008). A group intervention for parents and children achieved greater weight loss in obese children than routine care. *Evidence-Based Nursing, 11*, 43.

Mick, J. (2009). Men were surprised by the severity of symptoms they experienced after laparoscopic radical prostatectomy. *Evidence-Based Nursing, 12*(1), 28.

Nyamathi, A., Salem, B. E., Zhang, S., Farabee, D., Hall, B., Khalilifard, F., & Leake, B. (2015). Nursing case management, peer coaching, and hepatitis A and B vaccine completion among homeless men recently released on parole. *Nursing Research, 64*(3), 177-189.

Stein, J., & Levitt, M. A. (2003). A randomized, controlled double-blind trial of usual-dose versus high-dose albuterol via continuous nebulization in patients with acute bronchospasm. *Annals of Emergency Medicine, 10*(1), 31-36.

Taylor, G. W., Pritzel, S. J., Manz, M. C., Borgnakke, W. S., Eber, R. M., & Bouman, P. D. (2005). Frequency of dental prophylaxis and glycemic control in type 2 diabetes. *Journal of Dental Hygiene, 79*(4), 22-25.

Turner-Sack, A. M., Menna, R, Setchell, S. R., Maan, C., Cataudella, D. (2016). Psychological functioning, post-traumatic growth, and coping in parents and siblings of adolescent cancer survivors. *Oncology Nursing Forum, 43*(1), 48-56.

Yost, J. (2007). Intranasal fentanyl and intravenous morphine did not differ for pain relief in children with closed long-bone fractures. *Evidence-Based Nursing, 11*(2), 42.

Ziegler, E. E., Nelson, S. E., & Jeter, J. M. (2009). Iron status of breastfed infants is improved equally by medicinal iron and iron-fortified cereal. *American Journal of Clinical Nutrition, 90*(1), 76-87.

3 Gathering and Appraising the Literature

INTRODUCTION

The phrases *literature review* or *review of the literature* refer to a key step in the research process for researchers, as well as for consumers of research. For researchers, the *literature review* is the section of a research study in which the researcher retrieves, critically appraises, and synthesizes previously existing knowledge. It is this literature review that is then used as the basis for the development of research questions and hypotheses by the researcher. Similarly, as consumers of research, nurses involved in evidence-based practice are also responsible for *reviewing the literature.* They systematically gather, critically appraise, and synthesize the best-available evidence to establish its strength, quality, and consistency to determine its applicability to practice. This chapter will help you learn more about how to critique the literature review performed by researchers and how to conduct an effective search of the literature and critically read, appraise, and synthesize sources as a consumer of research to address clinical questions.

LEARNING OUTCOMES

On completion of this chapter, you should be able to do the following:

- Discuss the purpose of a literature review in a research study.
- Discuss the purpose of reviewing the literature for an evidence-based and quality improvement project.
- Differentiate the purposes of a literature review from the evidence-based practice and the research perspective.
- Differentiate between primary and secondary sources.
- Differentiate between systematic reviews/meta-analyses and preappraised synopses.
- Discuss the purpose of reviewing the literature for developing evidence-based practice and quality improvement projects.
- Use the PICO format to guide a search of the literature.
- Conduct an effective search of the literature.
- Apply critiquing criteria for the evaluation of literature reviews in research studies.
- Critically read, appraise, and synthesize sources used to develop a literature review.

Activity 1

Sometimes it is difficult to understand the distinction between primary and secondary sources of information. A comparison that is always helpful is if you are considering giving a patient an injection for pain, whose report would you feel most comfortable evaluating—the report of a family member or nurse's aide (i.e., secondary source) or the report by the patient (i.e., primary source)? As a consumer of nursing research, you will also need to evaluate the credibility of literature in part on whether it is generated from primary or secondary sources so that you know whether you are reading a firsthand report or someone else's interpretation of the material. Below is a selected list of references from the study by Turner-Sack et al. (2016) (Appendix D in the textbook). Next to each reference, indicate whether it is a primary *(P)* or secondary *(S)* source. It may be helpful to retrieve the abstract or full text of the reference and refer to Table 3-1 in your textbook.

1. ________ Brown, R. T., Madan-Swain, A., & Lambert, R. (2003). Posttraumatic stress symptoms in adolescent survivors of childhood cancer and their mothers. *Journal of Traumatic Stress, 16*(4), 309-318. doi:10.1023/A:1024465415620

2. ________ Cordova, M. J., Cunningham, L. L., Carlson, C. R., & Andrykowski, M. A. (2001). Posttraumatic growth following breast cancer: A controlled comparison study. *Health Psychology, 20*(3), 176-185. doi:10.1037/0278-6133.20.3.176

3. ________ Tedeschi, R., Park, C. L., & Calhoun, L. G. (1998). *Posttraumatic growth: Positive changes in the aftermath of crisis.* Mahwah, NJ: Lawrence Erlbaum Associates.

4. ________ Tedeschi, R. G., & Calhoun, L. G. (1996). The Post-Traumatic Growth Inventory: Measuring the positive legacy of trauma. *Journal of Traumatic Stress, 9*(3), 455-471. doi:10.1002/jts.2490090305

Activity 2

Typically a literature review consists of numerous journal articles. The focus of the literature review and search strategies differs between a researcher's perspective and an evidence-based practice or quality improvement perspective. For each of the following statements, determine from which of these perspectives best describes a review of the literature:

A. A research perspective
B. An evidence-based practice or quality improvement perspective

1. ________ Review of literature helps to develop or refine a clinical question.
2. ________ Review of literature uses a problem/patient population, intervention, comparison, outcome (PICO) format to search the literature for the "best available evidence" to answer a clinical question.
3. ________ Review of literature helps to choose a design, sampling strategy, data collection, setting, instruments, and data analysis.
4. ________ Focus of review is critical appraisal of research, systematic reviews, practice guidelines, and other relevant documents.
5. ________ Uses review of literature to interpret and discuss study findings, draw conclusions, identify limitations, and suggest future studies.
6. ________ Uses review of literature to test research questions or hypotheses.

Activity 3

Although there are books, journals, and additional literature that remain available only in print versions located in libraries, many researchers and consumers of research conduct reviews of the literature using online bibliographic and abstract databases. The key to using these tools efficiently is understanding Boolean operators. For the following questions, choose the best operator to retrieve relevant information from a database.

a. Not
b. Or
c. And

1. ________ A student wants to better understand first-time attempt NLCEX pass rates. The student wants to find studies that focused on degree programs (both baccalaureate and associate). The search terms are "education, nursing, associate" and "education, nursing, baccalaureate." Which Boolean operator would best focus the search?
2. ________ The student wants to exclude studies that included diploma programs. Which operator would the student add before the search terms "education, nursing, diploma programs"?
3. ________ The student did not find many articles using both baccalaureate and associate degree programs. Which operator would include a more comprehensive set of articles that included these search terms?

Activity 4

Match the definition in Column A with the appropriate term in Column B

Column A

1. ________ A scholarly journal that uses a panel of internal and external reviewers to review submitted manuscripts for publication; uses specific criteria to determine if manuscripts should be published
2. ________ Systematic and critical appraisal of the most important literature on a topic
3. ________ May include committee reports, policy documents, or dissertations
4. ________ Used to define the relationships between words or groups of words in literature searches
5. ________ Software that formats citations
6. ________ Scholarly literature written by the person(s) who developed the theory or conducted the research
7. ________ Commentary about a publication's strengths, weaknesses, applicability to a patient population, and potential relevance
8. ________ Terms indexers have assigned to articles in a database; can help you to match terms in a search to those terms specifically used in a database
9. ________Include CINAHL, Medline, Cochrane Database of Systematic Reviews
10. ________ Scholarly literature written by person(s) other than the individual who developed a theory or conducted the research; may be a response, summary, or critique of another's work
11. ________ A search using relevant databases in addition to CINAHL PLUS with full text via EBSCO, and MEDLINE via Ovid; search makes use of key MESH terms and Boolean logic (AND, OR, NOT) to address a clinical question
12. ________ Software program used to connect with the World Wide Web; examples include Internet Explorer, Chrome, Safari)

Column B

a. Gray literature
b. Web browser
c. Peer-reviewed journal
d. Primary source
e. Secondary source
f. Electronic search
g. Literature review
h. Electronic database
i. Boolean operator
j. Controlled vocabulary
k. Citation management software
l. Preappraised synopses

POSTTEST

Refer to the study by Nyamathi et al. (2015) (Appendix A in the textbook) to answer the following questions.

1. What level of evidence does this study provide?
   a. Level I
   b. Level II
   c. Level III
   d. Level IV
   e. Level V
   f. A single study cannot provide a level of evidence.

For questions 2 through 4, use the following references from Nyamathi et al. (2016) in Appendix A. It may be helpful to look up the references and journal information.

1. Hunt, D. R., & Saab, S. (2009). Viral hepatitis in incarcerated adults: A medical and public health concern. *American Journal of Gastroenterology, 104,* 1024-1031. doi:10.1038/ajg.2008.143
2. Lazarus, R. S., & Folkman, S. (1984). *Stress, appraisal, and coping.* New York, NY: Springer.
3. Nyamathi, A., Christiani, A., Nahid, P., Gregerson, P., & Leake, B. (2006). A randomized controlled trial of two treatment programs for homeless adults with latent tuberculosis infection. *International Journal of Tuberculosis and Lung Disease, 10,* 775-782.

4. Centers for Disease Control and Prevention. (2010). *Table 2.1 reported cases of acute hepatitis A by state—United States, 2006–2010.*
   Atlanta, GA: U.S. Department of Health and Human Services. Retrieved from http://www.cdc.gov/hepatitis/Statistics/2010Surveillance/Table2.1.htm
5. Zuckerman, A. J. (1996). Chapter 70: Hepatitis viruses. In S. Baron (Ed.), *Medical microbiology* (4th ed.). Galveston, TX: University of Texas Medical Branch.

2. For each of the previous references, indicate whether it is:
   a. Primary (*P*) source
   b. Secondary (*S*) source
   c. Gray literature

   1. ______________________________
   2. ______________________________
   3. ______________________________
   4. ______________________________
   5. ______________________________

3. For each of the previous references, determine if the source is
   a. Peer-reviewed
   b. Nonrefereed

   1. ______________________________
   2. ______________________________
   3. ______________________________
   4. ______________________________
   5. ______________________________

4. Does the literature review (A) identify research questions and hypotheses or (B) answer a clinical question?

5. Where can you find the purpose of the study?
   a. Literature review

   b. Theoretical framework

   c. Purpose

   d. Methods

   e. Discussion

6. Rewrite the following objectives as a PICO question:
"The study focused on completion of the HAV and HBV vaccine series among homeless men on parole. The efficacy of three levels of peer coaching (PC) and nurse-delivered interventions was compared at 12-month follow-up: (a) intensive peer coaching and nurse case management; (b) intensive peer coaching intervention condition, with minimal nurse involvement; and (c) usual care intervention condition, which included minimal peer coaching and nurse involvement."

P ____

I ____

C ____

O ____

7. Do the authors use theoretical/conceptual sources?
   a. Yes
   b. No

8. How is the literature review organized?
   a. Chronologically

   b. By concept or variables

   c. Alphabetically by author

   d. By level of evidence

REFERENCES

Brown, R. T., Madan-Swain, A., & Lambert, R. (2003). Posttraumatic stress symptoms in adolescent survivors of childhood cancer and their mothers. *Journal of Traumatic Stress, 16*(4), 309-318. doi:10.1023/A:1024465415620

Centers for Disease Control and Prevention. (2010). *Table 2.1 reported cases of acute hepatitis A by state—United States, 2006-2010.* Atlanta, GA: U.S. Department of Health and Human Services. Retrieved from http://www.cdc.gov/hepatitis/Statistics/2010Surveillance/Table2.1.htm

Cordova, M. J., Cunningham, L. L., Carlson, C. R., & Andrykowski, M. A. (2001). Posttraumatic growth following breast cancer: A controlled comparison study. *Health Psychology, 20*(3), 176-185. doi:10.1037/0278-6133.20.3.176

Hunt, D. R., & Saab, S. (2009). Viral hepatitis in incarcerated adults: A medical and public health concern. *American Journal of Gastroenterology, 104,* 1024-1031. doi:10.1038/ajg.2008.143

Lazarus, R. S., & Folkman, S. (1984). *Stress, appraisal, and coping.* New York, NY: Springer.

Nyamathi, A., Salem, B. E., Zhang, S., Farabee, D., Hall, B., Khalilifard, F., & Leake, B. (2015). Nursing case management, peer coaching, and hepatitis A and B vaccine completion among homeless men recently released on parole. *Nursing Research, 64*(3), 177-189.

Nyamathi, A., Christiani, A., Nahid, P., Gregerson, P., & Leake, B. (2006). A randomized controlled trial of two treatment programs for homeless adults with latent tuberculosis infection. *International Journal of Tuberculosis and Lung Disease, 10,* 775-782.

Tedeschi, R., Park, C. L., & Calhoun, L. G. (1998). *Posttraumatic growth: Positive changes in the aftermath of crisis.* Mahwah, NJ: Lawrence Erlbaum Associates.

Tedeschi, R. G., & Calhoun, L. G. (1996). The Post-Traumatic Growth Inventory: Measuring the positive legacy of trauma. *Journal of Traumatic Stress, 9*(3), 455-471. doi:10.1002/jts.2490090305

Turner-Sack, A. M., Menna, R., Setchell, S. R., Maan, C., & Cataudella, D. (2016). Psychological functioning, post traumatic growth, and coping in parents and siblings of adolescent cancer survivors. *Oncology Nursing Forum, 43*(1), 48-56.

Zuckerman, A. J. (1996). Chapter 70: Hepatitis viruses. In S. Baron (Ed.), *Medical microbiology* (4th ed.). Galveston, TX: University of Texas Medical Branch.

4 Theoretical Frameworks for Research

INTRODUCTION

It is not uncommon for beginning consumers of research to find the theoretical part of a study to be their least favorite component. However, nursing science is the result of the interchange between research and theory. This chapter provides an overview of the use of theoretical frameworks for nursing research. An understanding of theoretical frameworks will help you examine the logical, consistent link among the theoretical framework, concepts in the study, and methods of measurement.

LEARNING OUTCOMES

On completion of this chapter, you should be able to do the following:

- Describe the relationships among theory, research, and practice.
- Identify the purpose of conceptual and theoretical frameworks for nursing research.
- Differentiate between conceptual and operational definitions.
- Identify the different types of theories used in nursing research.
- Describe how a theory or conceptual framework guides research.
- Explain the points of critical appraisal used to evaluate the appropriateness, cohesiveness, and consistency of a framework guiding research.

Activity 1

Place the steps a researcher must address when deciding to study a concept or construct in order.

A. Determine a method to measure or quantify a concept/construct.
B. Precisely and explicitly describe and explain the concept.
C. Devise a mechanism to identify and confirm the presence of the concept of interest.

________, ________, ________.

Activity 2

Match the definition in Column A with the appropriate term in Column B.

Column A

1. ________ A graphic or symbolic representation of a phenomenon that assists the reader to visualize the key concepts or constructs and their identified interrelationships
2. ________ A complex concept that usually is composed of more than one concept that is built or constructed to fit a purpose
3. ________ Set of interrelated concepts that provides a systematic view of a phenomenon
4. ________ Image or symbolic representation of an abstract idea
5. ________ Defines what instruments will be used to assess the presence of the concepts and will be used to describe the amount or degree to which the concept exists
6. ________ Goes beyond the general language meaning found in the dictionary to define or explain the meaning of a concept
7. ________ May also be called a theoretical framework; a set of interrelated concepts that represents an image of a phenomenon

Column B

a. Theory
b. Concept
c. Conceptual definition
d. Operational definition
e. Model
f. Construct
g. Conceptual framework

Activity 3

The theories developed specifically by and for nurses can be classified into three categories: (A) situation-specific theory, (B) middle range theory, (C) grand theory. Place the theories in order of *most* abstract to *least* abstract.

1. ______________________, ______________________, ______________________

Identify the category of theory for each of the following using the three categories listed earlier.

2. The Behavioral Systems Model (Johnson, D. E., 1990) ______________________
3. Becoming a Mother (Mercer, R. T., 2004) ______________________
4. Theory of Resilience (Polk, L. V., 1997) ______________________
5. Notes on Nursing (Nightingale, F., 1969, 1860) ______________________

Activity 4

In nursing research, theories are used in the research process. Identify the ways in which theories are used in the research process using *true* (T) or *false* (F).

1. Theory is generated as the outcome of a research study. ________
2. Theories can be tested by research but not by practice. ________
3. Nursing knowledge is built on the foundation of practice, theory, and research, and all are interwoven. ________
4. Theories cannot be used to predict or explain another phenomenon. ________
5. Theories from other disciplines cannot be used as a foundation for research or practice in nursing. ________
6. Nurses shouldn't use theories because nursing is a practice discipline. ________
7. Evidence-based nursing care is based on an understanding of relationships between concepts and phenomena. ________

Activity 5

In a study to test a theory, researchers follow certain steps. Put the following steps in sequential order from 1 (first step) to 4 (last step).

a. ________ Interprets the findings considering the predictive ability of the theory

b. ________ Chooses a theory of interest and selects a propositional statement to be examined

c. ________ Determines if there are implications for further use of the theory in practice

d. ________ Develops hypotheses that have measurable variables

POSTTEST

Nursing theories have similarities and differences based on their scope or degree of abstraction. For questions 1 through 8, match the description in Column A with the appropriate type of nursing theory in Column B. (The type of nursing theories in Column B are used more than once, and more than one can apply to the description in Column A.)

Column A

1. _______ Composed of a limited number of concepts
2. _______ Sometimes referred to as *conceptual models*
3. _______ Focused on a limited aspect of reality
4. _______ Narrow in scope
5. _______ Most abstract level of theory
6. _______ All-inclusive conceptual structures that tend to include views on the person, health, and the environment
7. _______ Explains a small aspect of phenomena and processes
8. _______ Usually limited to specific populations or a field of practice

Column B

a. Grand
b. Situation-specific
c. Middle range

For questions 9 through 15, answer *true* (T) or *false* (F).

9. _______ Use of nonnursing theories is not important for providing evidence-based care.
10. _______ Correlational research designs are often used in studies that use a theory as a framework for a study.
11. _______ Beginning with theory gives a researcher a logical way of collecting data to describe, explain, and predict nursing practice.
12. _______ Certain grand theories are better than others with respect to nursing research.
13. _______ Qualitative research designs are used to test a theory.
14. _______ Theories are only used in qualitative research designs.
15. _______ Theory-generating research is inductive; it uses a process by which generalizations are developed from specific observations.

REFERENCES

Johnson, D. E. (1990). The behavioral system model for nursing. In M. E. Parker (Ed.), *Nursing theories in practice* (pp. 23-32). New York, NY: National League for Nursing Press.

Mercer, R. T. (2004). Becoming a mother versus maternal role attainment. *Journal of Nursing Scholarship*, *36*(3), 226-232.

Nightingale, F. (1969). *Notes on nursing: what it is and what it is not.* New York, NY: Dover Publications (Original work published 1860).

Polk, L. V. (1997). Toward a middle range theory of resilience. *Advances in Nursing Science, 19*(3), 1-13.

5 Introduction to Qualitative Research

INTRODUCTION

Qualitative research is a term often applied to naturalistic investigations—research that involves studying phenomena in places where they are occurring. Qualitative research approaches are based on a perceived perspective or holistic worldview that says there is not a single reality. Instead, reality is viewed as based on perceptions that differ from person to person and change over time; meaning can only be truly understood if it is associated with a specific situation or context. Qualitative research is about understanding phenomena and finding meaning through examining the pieces that make up the whole. Through different forms of qualitative nursing research methods, each method of investigation presents a unique approach to studying the phenomena of interest to nurses and the discipline.

Evidence-based practice has been primarily focused on findings that come from systematic reviews of the literature that use models examining the effectiveness of interventions. As acceptance has grown for the use of evidence-based practice in nursing, arguments about the place of qualitative research in this process have arisen. Questions of interest to nursing that have not been previously or thoroughly studied are often best investigated using qualitative methods. When new perspectives are introduced to practice, the use of qualitative investigation may be the best way to gain early understanding that can later be studied using empirical measures. However, reviews of qualitative research about a given topic can also provide meaningful insight into practice issues that can be directly applied in clinical settings.

LEARNING OUTCOMES

On completion of this chapter, you should be able to do the following:

- Describe the components of a qualitative research report.
- Describe the beliefs generally held by qualitative researchers.
- Identify four ways qualitative findings can be used in evidence-based practice.

Activity 1

Chapter 5 of the textbook provides an overview of qualitative research and introduces a variety of terms that have important implications for understanding qualitative research. Take some time to define the following terms and be sure that you can differentiate them.

Column A

1. ________ Overarching, broad categories of meaning
2. ________ Where people live every day—homes, schools, communities
3. ________ Nonprobability sampling in which a researcher selects participants considered typical of the population
4. ________ Point where enough data have been collected that the information being shared becomes repetitive; no new ideas are emerging
5. ________ Observation is defined by its circumstance or context
6. ________ Philosophical beliefs or worldview
7. ________ Places where participants are recruited and data are collected
8. ________ Finding and engaging participants in the research
9. ________ Broad interview question that seeks the "big picture"
10. ________ Characteristics that limit the population to a homogeneous group of participants

Column B

A. Naturalistic settings
B. Context dependent
C. Purposive sample
D. Recruitment
E. Data saturation
F. Setting
G. Themes
H. Paradigm
I. Inclusion and exclusion criteria
J. Grand Tour question

Activity 2

Compare qualitative research with quantitative research for the following steps in the research process. Place the following descriptions where they belong in the table:

a. Statistics and numbers
b. Until data saturation
c. Naturalistic setting, numbers
d. Predetermined number of participants

	Qualitative	Quantitative
Sample recruitment		
Data collection		

Activity 3

Review Appendix C (van Dijk et al., 2016). Find and summarize the following elements.

	Element	Summary
Purpose		
Method		
Sample and setting		
Data collection		

POSTTEST

1. Identify whether each of the following beliefs reflects the quantitative or qualitative research method.

   a. ________ Statistical explanation

   b. ________ Interviews

   c. ________ Multiple realities

   d. ________ Naturalistic setting

   e. ________ Predetermined number of participants

   f. ________ Quotations

2. Put the following components of a qualitative research report in sequential order from 1 (first step) to 7 (last step) and provide a brief description of each.

   ________ Data analysis:

   ________ Sample:

   ________ Review of the literature:

   ________ Data collection:

   ________ Study setting:

   ________ Findings:

   ________ Study design:

REFERENCE

van Dijk, J. F. M., Vervoort, Sigrid C. J. M., van Wijck, A. J. M., Kalkman, C. J., & Schuurmans, M. J. (2016). Postoperative patients' perspective on rating pain: A qualitative study. *International Journal of Nursing Studies, 53*, 260-269.

6 Qualitative Approaches to Research

INTRODUCTION

Qualitative research continues to gain recognition as a sound method for investigating the complex human phenomena less easily explored using quantitative methods. Qualitative research methods provide ways to address both the science and art of nursing. Qualitative methods are especially well suited to address phenomena related to health and illness that are of interest to nurses and nursing practice. Nurse researchers and investigators from other disciplines are continuing to discover the value of findings obtained through qualitative studies. Nurses can be better prepared to critique the appropriateness of a research design and identify the usefulness of the study findings when the unique differences between quantitative and qualitative research approaches are understood.

Although there are many designs for qualitative research, five methods are most commonly used by nurses. These methods are phenomenology, grounded theory, ethnography, case study, and historical. A newer methodology known as *community-based participatory research* that is gaining increased respect from nursing scientists who are investigating behavioral phenomena is also described in this chapter. Understanding and care are concepts related to behaviors that are important to nurses in the practice of clinical nursing care in a variety of settings across the lifespan. Each of these qualitative methods allows the researcher to approach the phenomenon of interest from a different perspective. Each offers the investigator a different perspective and suggests findings that address different realms of human experience.

LEARNING OUTCOMES

On completion of this chapter, you should be able to do the following:

- Identify the processes of phenomenological, grounded theory, ethnographic, and case study methods.
- Recognize appropriate use of community-based participatory research methods.
- Discuss significant issues that arise in conducting qualitative research in relation to such topics as ethics, criteria for judging scientific rigor, and combination of research methods.
- Apply critiquing criteria to evaluate a report of qualitative research.

Activity 1

Match the following definitions in Column A with the appropriate terms in Column B.

Column A

1. ________ No new data emerging
2. ________ Select experiences to help the researcher test ideas and gather complete information about developing concepts
3. ________ Outsider's view
4. ________ Identify personal biases about the phenomenon
5. ________ Insider's view
6. ________ Symbolic categories that include smaller categories
7. ________ Individuals who have special knowledge, status, or communication skills and who are willing to teach the ethnographer about the phenomenon

Column B

a. Theoretical sampling
b. Emic
c. Etic
d. Data saturation
e. Bracketed
f. Domains
g. Key informants

Activity 2

Six qualitative research methods are discussed in the textbook in relation to five basic research elements. Use your textbook to compare research elements of each of the different types of qualitative methods. Find the brief description of key aspects of each element for the different qualitative methods. This activity will assist you to compare and contrast the similarities and differences in these methods. Use the following research methods to complete Tables 1 to 5.

A. Phenomenology
B. Grounded theory
C. Ethnography
E. Case study
F. Community-based participatory research

1. Identifying the phenomenon	
1. ____________	A study to systematically assess the voice of a community to plan context-appropriate action
2. ____________	Study of day-to-day existence for a particular group of people
3. ____________	Study of the description and interpretation of cultural or social groups and systems
4. ____________	A focus on an individual, family, community, an organization, or some other complex phenomenon
5. ____________	Interested in social processes from perspective of human interactions or patterns of action and interaction between and among various types of social units

2. Structuring the study	
1. ____________	Asks about the lived experience. The research perspective is bracketed. The sample has either lived in the past or is living the experience being investigated.
2. ____________	Questions are about lifeways or patterns of behavior within a social context of a culture or subculture. The researcher attempts to make sense of the world from an insider's point of view. The sample often consists of key informants who have special knowledge, status, or communication skills and who are willing to teach the researcher about the phenomenon of interest.
3. ____________	Questions address basic social processes and tend to be action oriented. The researcher brings some knowledge of the literature, but exhaustive review is not done before beginning the research. The sample are participants who are experiencing the circumstance and selecting events or incidents related to the social processes being studied.
4. ____________	Assumes that a phenomenon may be separated from its context. Researchers recognize that engaging members of the study population as active and equal participants, in all phases of research, is crucial.
5. ____________	Questions about issues that serve as a foundation to uncover complexity and pursue understanding. The perspective of the researcher is reflected in the questions. Researchers may choose the most common cases or instead select the most unusual ones.

3. Data collection	
1. ____________	Uses interviews, observations, document reviews, and other methods.
2. ____________	Engages stakeholders in discovering the answers to the community problems.
3. ____________	Written or oral data may be collected.
4. ____________	Data are collected through interviews and skilled observations of individuals interacting in a social setting.
5. ____________	Involves participant observation, immersion, and informant interviews.

4. Data analysis	
1. ____________	Move from the participant's description to the researcher's synthesis of all participants' descriptions.
2. ____________	Data are often collected and analyzed simultaneously, reflecting and revising meanings.
3. ____________	This stage of research is the "think" phase and is where what has been learned is interpreted or analyzed. The research has the role of linking the ideas provided by the stakeholders in an understandable way so that evidence for specific ways to address the problem can be provided to the community group.
4. ____________	Data are collected and analyzed simultaneously, searching for meaning of cultural symbols in the informants' language.
5. ____________	Data collection and analysis occur simultaneously and involve use of theoretical sampling, constant comparative method, and axial coding.

5. Description of the findings	
1. ____________	Large quantities of data provide examples from the data and propositions about relationships of phenomena.
2. ____________	Information obtained in earlier research stages sets the stage for community planning, implementation, and evaluation.
3. ____________	Descriptive language and diagrams are used to show theory connections to the data.
4. ____________	Cases are chronologically developed, creating a story that describes case dimensions or vignettes that emphasize various aspects of the case.
5. ____________	Involves a narrative elaboration of the lived experience.

Activity 3

The five qualitative methods of research are the phenomenology, grounded theory, ethnographic, case study, and historical. For each characteristic listed here, indicate which method of qualitative research it describes. Use the abbreviations from the key provided. Some characteristics may be described by more than one method.

Key:

A = Phenomenology
B = Grounded theory
C = Ethnographic
D = Case study

1. ________ Uses "emic" and "etic" views of participants' worlds.
2. ________ Research questions focus on basic social processes that shape behavior.
3. ________ Central meanings arise from participants' descriptions of lived experience.
4. ________ Focuses on a dimension of day-to-day existence.
5. ________ Uses theoretical sampling to analyze data.
6. ________ Studies the peculiarities and commonalities of a specific case.
7. ________ Discovers "domains" to analyze data.
8. ________ States that individuals' history is a dimension of the present.
9. ________ Attempts to discover underlying social forces that shape human behavior.
10. ________ Attention is given to a single case.
11. ________ "Key informants" are interviewed.
12. ________ Focuses on describing cultural groups.
13. ________ Uses constant comparative method during data analysis.
14. ________ Researcher "brackets" personal bias or perspective.
15. ________ Can include quantitative and qualitative data.
16. ________ Participants are currently experiencing a circumstance.
17. ________ Collects remembered information from participants.
18. ________ Involves "field work."
19. ________ May use photographs to describe current behavioral practices.
20. ________ May not include exhaustive literature search.
21. ________ Uses an inductive approach to understanding basic social processes.

Activity 4

Read the Methods section of the study by van Dijk et al. (2016) in Appendix C of the textbook and answer the following questions.

1. What research design was used to conduct this research study?
   a. Case study
   b. Grounded theory
   c. Meta-summary
   d. Phenomenological method
   e. Mixed methods

2. Describe the sample in this study.
   a. Emic
   b. Etic
   c. Snowball
   d. Purposive

3. What important procedures and methods were used to collect data in this study?
   a. Semistructured in-depth interviews, audiotaped and transcribed
   b. Demographic questionnaire
   c. Skilled observation
   d. Immersion in the sample setting, observation, and interviews

4. Which of the following methods were used during data analysis? (Choose all that apply.)
   a. Research triangulation
   b. Axial coding
   c. Constant comparison analysis

POSTTEST

For questions 1 through 5, answer *true* (T) or *false* (F).

1. _______ Qualitative research focuses on the whole of human experience in naturalistic settings.

2. _______ *External criticism in historical research* refers to the authenticity of data sources.

3. _______ In qualitative research, one would expect the number of participants to be as large as those usually found in quantitative studies.

4. _______ The researcher is viewed as the major instrument for data collection.

5. _______ Qualitative studies strive to eliminate extraneous variables.

6. To what does the term *saturation* in qualitative research refer?
   a. Data repetition
   b. Participant exhaustion
   c. Researcher exhaustion
   d. Sample size

7. Data in qualitative research are often collected by which of the following procedures?
   a. Questionnaires sent out to participants
   b. Observation of participants in naturalistic settings
   c. Interviews
   d. All of the above

8. The qualitative method that includes an inductive approach using a systematic set of procedures to create a theory about basic social processes is known as which of the following?
   a. Phenomenology
   b. Grounded theory
   c. Ethnography
   d. Case study
   e. Community-based participatory research

9. What is the qualitative method that attempts to construct the meaning of the lived experience of human phenomena?
   a. Phenomenology
   b. Grounded theory
   c. Ethnography
   d. Case study
   e. Community-based participatory research

10. What qualitative research method would be most appropriate for studying the impact of culture on the health behaviors of urban Hispanic youth?
    a. Phenomenology
    b. Grounded theory
    c. Ethnography
    d. Case study
    e. Community-based participatory research

11. What qualitative method would be most appropriate for studying a family's experience with cystic fibrosis?
    a. Phenomenology
    b. Grounded theory
    c. Ethnography
    d. Case study
    e. Community-based participatory research

12. What qualitative method would you use to study the spread of HIV/AIDS in an urban area?
    a. Phenomenology
    b. Grounded theory
    c. Ethnography
    d. Case study
    e. Community-based participatory research

13. Which data analysis process is *not* used with grounded theory methodology?
    a. Bracketing
    b. Axial coding
    c. Theoretical sampling
    d. Open coding

REFERENCE

van Dijk, J. F. M., Vervoort, Sigrid C. J. M., van Wijck, A. J. M., Kalkman, C. J., & Schuurmans, M. J. (2016). Postoperative patients' perspective on rating pain: A qualitative study. *International Journal of Nursing Studies, 53*, 260-269.

7 Appraising Qualitative Research

INTRODUCTION

Qualitative research provides an opportunity to generate new knowledge about phenomena less easily studied with empirical or quantitative methods. Nurse researchers are increasingly using qualitative methods to explore holistic aspects less easily investigated with objective measures. In qualitative research, the data are less likely to involve numbers and most likely will include text derived from interviews, focus groups, observation, field notes, or other methods. The data tend to be mostly narrative or written words that require content rather than statistical analysis. The important contributions being made to nursing knowledge through qualitative studies make it important for nurses to possess skills that enable them to evaluate and critique qualitative research reports. This chapter describes the criteria needed to evaluate and critique qualitative research reports. Published research reports, whether they are quantitative or qualitative, must be viewed by the reviewers as having scientific merit, demonstrate rigor in the research conducted, present new knowledge, and be of interest to the journal's readers.

LEARNING OUTCOMES

On completion of this chapter, you should be able to do the following:

- Understand the role of critical appraisal in research and evidence-based practice.
- Identify the criteria for critiquing a qualitative research study.
- Identify the stylistic considerations in a qualitative study.
- Apply critical reading skills to the appraisal of qualitative research.
- Evaluate the strengths and weaknesses of a qualitative study.
- Describe the applicability of the findings of a qualitative study.
- Construct a written critique of a qualitative research report.

Activity 1

Critiquing qualitative research enables the nurse to make sense out of the research report, build on the body of knowledge about human phenomena, and consider how the knowledge might be applicable to nursing. Learning and applying a critiquing process is the first step in this process. Column A provides examples of information from the study by van Dijk et al. (2016) found in Appendix C of the textbook. Match the information in Column A with the appropriate qualitative critical appraisal criteria in Column B. Some of the criteria in Column B are used more than once.

Column A

1. ________ "From the analysis, three main themes emerged regarding the process of scoring one's pain experience: score-related factors, interpersonal factors, and the anticipated consequences of rating one's pain with an NRS score."
2. ________ "The questions were open-ended, and all interviews started with, 'The nurse regularly asks you to assign a number from 0 to 10 to your pain, where 0 is no pain and 10 is the "worst imaginable" pain. We heard from some patients that they perceived it as difficult to assign a number to their pain. How is that for you?'"
3. ________ "A qualitative approach according to grounded theory was used."
4. ________ "First the texts were read out in full to obtain an overall picture and then reread to elucidate the details. During open coding meaningful paragraphs were analyzed and initial concepts identified leading to fragmentation of the data."
5. ________ "Patients were selected purposively by the researcher and to create a diverse sample patients were selected with regard to sex, age, ethnicity, previous pain experiences, and previous experience with rating an NRS score. Theoretical sampling was used as much as possible: we started with a homogeneous sample of patients, and as the data collection proceeded and themes emerged, we turned to a more heterogeneous sample to see under what conditions the themes hold."
6. ________ "The aim of this qualitative study was to explore how patients assign a number on the basis of the NRS to their currently experienced postoperative pain and which considerations influence this process."
7. ________ "Although our study was restricted to only one university hospital, the richness of the data makes us confident that our analysis has captured the most typical aspects of patients; underlying process for rating their pain on the NRS."
8. ________ "The theoretical model in development was compared with the interview transcripts to verify the interpretation into the original interview texts."
9. ________ "For optimal pain treatment, patients and professionals must communicate effectively and have a shared understanding of the burden of the patient's currently experienced pain."
10. ________ "Several patients said that everyone experiences pain differently and therefore will assign their own value from 0 to 10. 'It is difficult to measure. You've got your interpretation and I've got mine' (male, age 51)."
11. ________ "Knowledge of the factors in this study that influence a patient's pain scoring can help professionals use simple questions to explore patients' unique pain experiences and consequently titrate analgesic treatment in dialogue with the patient, improving the quality and safety of care."
12. ________ "Interviews were conducted in a private room on the ward, digitally recorded and transcribed verbatim."

Column B

a. Statement of phenomenon of interest
b. Purpose
c. Method
d. Sampling
e. Data collection
f. Data analysis
g. Findings
h. Discussion/conclusions/implications/recommendations

Activity 2

The textbook discusses overall purposes of qualitative research. Identify the purposes of qualitative research that the textbook identifies; mark each of the following as *true* (T) or *false* (F).

1. ________ Qualitative research provides the opportunity to give voice to those who have been disenfranchised and have no history.
2. ________ Qualitative research creates solutions to practical problems.
3. ________ Qualitative research initiates the examination of important concepts in nursing practice, education, or administration.
4. ________ Qualitative research discovers evidence about a phenomenon of interest that can lead to instrument development.

Activity 3

When critiquing a qualitative study, the following are important components of the analysis of data. Identify the following as a component of (A) credibility, (B) auditability, or (C) fittingness.

1. ________ Can be confirmed when others, not engaged in the research, are able to follow the audit trail of the primary researchers.
2. ________ Can be confirmed when the informants recognize the reported findings as their personal experience.
3. ________ A research process that allows the work of a qualitative researcher or a person critiquing a research report to follow the thinking and/or conclusions of a researcher.
4. ________ "Are the findings applicable outside the study?"
5. ________ "Are the results or feelings meaningful to people not involved in the research?"
6. ________ Qualitative research steps taken to ensure the accuracy, validity, and soundness of the data.
7. ________ "Are the findings meaningful to others who are in similar situations?"
8. ________ Is confirmed when the reader is provided with an opportunity to determine the usefulness of the data outside the study.

POSTTEST

For questions 1 through 5, answer *true* (T) or *false* (F).

1. ________ Unlike quantitative research, prediction and control of phenomena are not the aim of qualitative research.
2. ________ Quotations are not an effective way to help the reader understand the insider's view.
3. ________ The goal of a published qualitative research study is to describe in as much detail as possible the insider's view of the phenomenon being studied.
4. ________ In a qualitative study, you should expect to find hypotheses.
5. ________ Page limitations for publishing a research study are not imposed by journals.

For questions 6 through 9, match the term in Column B with the appropriate definition in Column A.

Column A	Column B
6. ______ A process in which the researcher identifies personal biases about the phenomenon of interest to clarify how personal experience and beliefs may color what is heard and reported.	a. Phenomena
7. ______ Things that are perceived by our senses.	b. Bracketing
8. ______ A point when data collection can cease. It occurs when the information being shared with the researcher becomes repetitive.	c. Saturation
9. ______ A label that represents a way of describing large quantities of data in a condensed format.	d. Theme

REFERENCE

van Dijk, J. F. M., Vervoort, Sigrid C. J. M., van Wijck, A. J. M., Kalkman, C. J., & Schuurmans, M. J. (2016). Postoperative patients' perspective on rating pain: A qualitative study. *International Journal of Nursing Studies, 53*, 260-269.

8 Introduction to Quantitative Research

INTRODUCTION

The phrase *research design* is used to describe the overall plan of a particular study. The design is the researcher's plan for answering specific research questions in the most accurate and efficient way possible. In quantitative research, the plan outlines how the hypotheses will be tested. The design ties together the present research problem, the knowledge of the past, and the implications for the future. Thus the choice of a design reflects the researcher's experience, expertise, knowledge, and biases.

LEARNING OUTCOMES

On completion of this chapter, you should be able to do the following:

- Define *research design.*
- Identify the purpose of a research design.
- Define *control* and *fidelity* as it affects research design and the outcomes of a study.
- Compare and contrast the elements that affect fidelity and control.
- Begin to evaluate what degree of control should be exercised in a study.
- Define *internal validity.*
- Identify threats to internal validity.
- Define *external validity.*
- Identify the conditions that affect external validity.
- Identify the links between the study design and evidence-based practice.
- Evaluate research design using critiquing questions.

Activity 1

Match the definitions in Column A with the research design terms in Column B. Check the glossary for help with terms.

Column A

1. ________ The antecedent variable
2. ________ Sampling selection in which each element has an equal chance for selection into the control or intervention group
3. ________ Methods to keep the study conditions constant during the study
4. ________ Methods to ensure that data collection procedures remain consistent for all participants
5. ________ The vehicle for hypothesis testing or answering research questions
6. ________ Small, preliminary study
7. ________ Degree to which the experimental conditions, and not uncontrolled factors, lead to the results of the study
8. ________ Degree to which the study results can be applied to the larger population
9. ________ Can reduce the credibility or dependability of the results of a study
10. ________ Group that receives the treatment in a study
11. ________ Presumed effect of the experimental variable on the outcome
12. ________ Comparison group

Column B

a. External validity
b. Internal validity
c. Bias
d. Research design
e. Control
f. Experimental group
g. Dependent variable
h. Independent variable
i. Control group
j. Pilot study
k. Constancy
l. Randomization

Activity 2

For each of the following situations, identify the type of threat to internal validity from Column A below. Then use Column B to suggest how the problem can be corrected.

Column A

a. History
b. Instrumentation
c. Maturation
d. Mortality
e. Selection bias
f. Testing

Column B

g. Use a short interval between the testing periods.
h. Use Solomon four-group design or use equivalent forms of the instrument.
i. Randomly assign participants to groups.
j. Data from some cohorts may be excluded from the analysis; if the whole sample was affected, the author should include this information in the study or may elect to redo the study.
k. Analyze the participants who remain in the study and those who dropped out to determine if there was a difference. Examine where the participants dropped out; for instance, did more participants drop out of the experimental group than the control group? Researchers may oversample to ensure that they will have an adequate sample even after attrition. They may also use a pilot study to determine if there is a factor in the experimental or control group that may lead to differential loss of participants.
l. Calibrate study equipment; or for observational data, use similar training for all data collectors.

1. ________, ________ The researcher tested the effectiveness of a new method of teaching drug dosage and solution calculations to nursing students using a standardized calculation exam at the beginning, midpoint, and end of a 2-week course.

2. ________, ________ In a study of the results of a hypertension teaching program conducted at a senior center, blood pressures taken by volunteers using their personal equipment were compared before and after the program.

3. ________, ________ A major increase in cigarette taxes occurs during a 1-year follow-up study of the impact of a smoking cessation program.

4. ________, ________ The smoking cessation rates of an experimental group consisting of volunteers for a smoking cessation program were compared with the results of a control group of people who wanted to quit on their own without a special program.

5. ________, ________ Thirty percent of the participants dropped out of an experimental study of the effect of a job-training program on employment for homeless women. More than 90% of the dropouts were single homeless women with at least two preschool-aged children, whereas the majority of participants successfully completing the program had no preschool-aged children.

6. ________, ________ Nurses on a maternity unit want to study the effect of a new hospital-based teaching program on mothers' confidence in caring for their newborn infants. A survey is mailed to participants by the researchers 1 month after discharge.

Activity 3

Research design is an all-encompassing term for the overall plan to answer the research questions, including the method and specific plans to control other factors that could influence the results of the study. To become acquainted with the major elements in the design of a study, match the parts of research design with the description in the left column. Answers may be used more than once.

Column A

_______ 1. Helps control threats to validity

_______ 2. Error, distortion of data analysis results

_______ 3. Measures (design, methods, analysis) that the researcher uses to hold conditions constant and avoid bias or error in the measurement of the dependent variable

_______ 4. Application of the outcome of the study to similar populations

_______ 5. Small study to test/refine data collection methods

_______ 6. Occurs between the independent variable and the dependent variable intervention fidelity

_______ 7. Controlled by homogeneous sample, consistent data collection, training and supervision of data collectors and/or interventionists, manipulation of the independent variable, randomization

_______ 8. Methods and procedures of data collection are the same for all participants

_______ 9. Helps determine sample size for a larger study

_______ 10. Maximizes results, decreases bias, controls preexisting conditions that may affect outcomes

Column B

a. Bias
b. Control
c. Intervening variable
d. Intervention fidelity
e. Generalizability
f. Pilot study
g. Constancy

Activity 4

Now that you are familiar with a research study, use the critiquing criteria in Chapter 8 in the textbook to critique the research design of the study by Nyamathi et al. (2015) (Appendix A in the text). Explain your answers.

1. Is the design appropriate?

2. Is the control consistent with the research design?

3. Think about the feasibility of this study. What are some of the feasibility challenges for this study?

4. Does the design logically flow from problem, framework, literature review, and hypothesis?

5. What are the threats to internal validity, and how did the investigators control for each?

6. What are the threats to external validity, and how did the investigators control for each?

Activity 5: Evidence-Based Practice Activity

Review the evidence-based practice tips from Chapter 8 in the textbook. Decide which of the following statements are likely *true* (T) or *false* (F), based on your reading.

1. ________ If a study discusses a population of interest to you in the literature review section but doesn't actually sample from your population of interest, the literature review of that study may be useful, however, the evidence from that study would not be useful for answering your evidence-based practice problem.

2. ________ The study you have selected tests an intervention. The authors describe using a randomized controlled trial design where all participants have an equal chance to be in the control or intervention group, a manual was created to train the interventionists for this study, and there was in-person training before the intervention started that included role playing; interventions were recorded and 25% of the recordings were reviewed by the study team to assess consistency. After the intervention, participants performed the skills taught in the intervention at the end of the teaching session and again after 3 months of performing the intervention independently. The authors do not describe specifically how they knew the participants had received and understood the treatment (a receipt). The authors demonstrated intervention fidelity and you could trust that the steps taken in the report were accurate.

3. ________ You read a study in your area of interest. The authors found that the intervention you are interested in did not produce a statistically significant result. You should not include this study in your evidence table.

4. ________ You are interested in a very specific subset of a population. You are unable to find any studies that specifically sample from your population. You cannot complete an evidence-based practice problem on this population.

POSTTEST

1. Fill in the blanks by selecting from the following list of terms. Not all terms will be used.

Constancy	Mortality
Control	Internal validity
Feasibility	External validity
Selection bias	Accuracy
Reliability	History
Maturation	

a. ________________________ is used to hold steady the conditions of the study.

b. ________________________ is used to describe that all aspects of a study logically follow from the problem statement.

c. The believability between this study and the world at large is known as ________________________.

d. The developmental, biological, or psychological processes known as ________________________ operate within a person over time and may influence the results of a study.

e. Time, participant availability, equipment, money, experience, and ethics are factors influencing the ________________________ of a study.

f. Selection bias, mortality, maturation, instrumentation, testing, and history influence the ________________________ of a study.

g. Voluntary (rather than random) assignment to an experimental or control condition creates a situation known as ________________________.

REFERENCES

Nyamathi, A., Salem, B., Zhang, S., Farabee, D., Hall, B., Khalilifard, F., & Leake, B. (2015). Nursing case management, peer coaching, and hepatitis A and B vaccine completion among homeless men recently released on parole: A randomized trial. *Nursing Research, 64*(3), 177-189.

9 Experimental and Quasi-Experimental Designs

INTRODUCTION

This chapter contains exercises for two categories of design: experimental and quasi-experimental. These types of designs allow researchers to test the effects of nursing actions and make statements about cause-and-effect relationships. Therefore they can be very helpful in testing solutions to nursing practice problems. However, a researcher chooses the design that allows a given situation or problem to be studied in the most accurate and effective way possible. Thus not all problems are amenable to immediate study by these two types of design. Rather, the choice of design is dependent on the development of knowledge relevant to the problem, plus the researcher's knowledge, experience, expertise, preferences, and resources.

LEARNING OUTCOMES

On completion of this chapter, you should be able to do the following:

- Describe the purpose of experimental and quasi-experimental research.
- Describe the characteristics of experimental and quasi-experimental designs.
- Distinguish between experimental and quasi-experimental designs.
- List the strengths and weaknesses of experimental and quasi-experimental designs.
- Identify the types of experimental and quasi-experimental designs.
- Identify potential internal and external validity issues associated with experimental and quasi-experimental designs.
- Critically evaluate the findings of experimental and quasi-experimental studies.
- Identify the contribution of experimental and quasi-experimental designs to evidence-based practice.

Activity 1

Fill in the blank for each of the following descriptions with a term selected from the list of types of experimental and quasi-experimental designs. Some terms may be used more than once and not all terms may be used.

After-only	One-group
After-only nonequivalent control group	Nonequivalent control group
Experimental	Solomon four-group
True experimental	Time series

1. ___________________ designs are particularly suitable for testing cause-and-effect relationships because they help eliminate potential alternative explanations (threats to validity) for the findings.
2. The type of design that has two groups identical to the true experimental design, plus an experimental after-group and a control after-group is known as a(n) ___________________ design.
3. A research approach used when only one group is available to study for trends over a longer period is called a(n) ___________________ design.
4. The ___________________ design is also known as the *post-test-only control group design* in which neither the experimental group nor the control group is pretested.
5. If a researcher wants to compare results obtained from an experimental group with a control group but was unable to conduct pretests or to randomly assign participants to groups, the study would be known as a(n) ___________________ design.
6. The ___________________ design includes three properties: randomization, control, and manipulation.

7. When participants are unable to be randomly assigned into experimental and control groups but are able to be pretested and posttested, the design is known as a(n) ___________________ design.

Activity 2

Review the study by Nyamathi et al. (2015) in Appendix A of the textbook, and then answer the following questions.

1. a. Did this study use a true experimental design? Yes or No ___________________

   b. Which of the following design elements were used in the study. Mark with an X all that were used.

   ________________________ This study had random assignment to groups and the group assignment was concealed.

   Processes used to maintain control:

   ________ Manipulation of the independent variable

   ________ Random assignment to group

   ________ Use of a control group

   ________ Preparation of intervention and data collection protocols

   ________ Manipulation, whereby different types of treatment were compared

2. A(n) ________ is the best way to test cause and effect because it allows the researcher to eliminate threats to internal validity.
   a. Time series
   b. After-only
   c. After-only nonequivalent control group
   d. Experimental

3. Which of the following conditions must be met to infer causality?
   a. The independent and dependent variables must be associated.
   b. The cause must precede the effect.
   c. The relationship must not be explained by another variable.
   d. Both A and B.
   e. All of the above.
   f. None of the above.

4. One important condition of experimental design is the relationship between the cause-and-effect variables. What are the independent variable(s)? Label each as *IV.* What are the dependent variable(s)? Label each as *DV.*

   a. ________ Usual care

   b. ________ Completion of the HAV and HBV vaccine series

   c. ________ Intensive peer coaching with minimal nurse-delivered interventions

   d. ________ Intensive peer coaching and nurse case management

Activity 3

The education department in a large hospital wants to test a program to educate and change nurses' attitudes regarding pain management. You have access to the following questionnaires: the Quick Pain Survey (QPS), the Pain Knowledge and Attitudes Questionnaire (PKQ), the Headache Assessment Tool (HAT), and the Survey on Pain in the Elderly (SPE). Your responsibility is to design a study to examine the outcome of this intervention program.

1. You decide to use a Solomon four-group design. Complete the chart below with an X to indicate which of the four groups receive the pretest and posttest pain questionnaire and which receive the experimental teaching program.

	Pretest	**Teaching**	**Posttest**
Group A	________	________	________
Group B	________	________	________
Group C	________	________	________
Group D	________	________	________

2. Pick the best method(s) to assign nurses to each of the four groups.
   a. Table of random numbers
   b. Assignment to group based on unit or geographical location
   c. Computerized random assignment
   d. Use two nonrandomly assigned groups and assume they are equivalent

3. What would you use as a pretest for the groups receiving the pretest?
   a. Quick Pain Survey (QPS)
   b. Pain Knowledge and Attitudes Questionnaire (PKQ)
   c. Headache Assessment Tool (HAT)
   d. Survey on Pain in the Elderly (SPE)
   e. Teaching program
   f. Nurses' attitudes

4. What is the experimental treatment?
   a. Quick Pain Survey (QPS)
   b. Pain Knowledge and Attitudes Questionnaire (PKQ)
   c. Headache Assessment Tool (HAT)
   d. Survey on Pain in the Elderly (SPE)
   e. Teaching program
   f. Nurses' attitudes

5. What is the outcome measure for each group?
   a. Quick Pain Survey (QPS)
   b. Pain Knowledge and Attitudes Questionnaire (PKQ)
   c. Headache Assessment Tool (HAT)
   d. Survey on Pain in the Elderly (SPE)
   e. Teaching program
   f. Nurses' attitudes

6. Based on your reading, for what types of issues is this design particularly effective?
   a. Reduces the effect of mortality on study results
   b. Allows the "standard treatment" group to receive the intervention after the first round of testing
   c. Allows nonrandom assignment to groups because of the larger number of groups
   d. Helpful in experimental studies in which the pretest might affect the outcome
   e. Both A and C
   f. Both B and D
   g. None of the above

7. What is the major advantage of this type of design?
   a. Allows the "standard treatment" group to receive the intervention after the first round of testing
   b. Effective in ruling out threats to internal validity that the before-and-after groups may experience.
   c. Allows nonrandom assignment to groups because of the larger number of groups
   d. Effective for highly sensitive issues, which might be affected by simply completing a questionnaire as a baseline pretest
   e. Both A and C
   f. Both B and D
   g. None of the above

8. What is a disadvantage of this type of design?
   a. A large number of participants must be available for assignment into the four groups.
   b. It requires a long time commitment from participants for multiple measures.
   c. Advanced statistical software is required.
   d. It allows increased threats to internal validity.
   e. Generalizability of results is decreased.

Activity 4

1. You may be questioning why anyone would use a quasi-experimental design if an experimental design has the advantage of being so much stronger in detecting cause-and-effect relationships and enabling the researcher to generalize the results to a wider population. Mark the instances where it might be advantageous to use a quasi-experimental design.

   ________ May be more practical

   ________ May be more feasible

   ________ May be more adaptable to real-world practice

   ________ May not be possible to randomly assign participants into groups for practical or ethical reasons

2. What must the researcher do to generalize the findings from a quasi-experimental research study?
   a. Carefully examine other factors that could account for differences between groups
   b. Ensure a large, randomly assigned sample
   c. Complete a thorough literature review that covers groups outside study population
   d. Work with ethics board to use disadvantaged populations

3. What must a clinician do before application of research findings into practice?
   a. Carefully critique the research study and also look for other factors, which might explain the results of the study.
   b. The results of the study must be evaluated to determine if other factors influenced the findings.
   c. The results should be compared with the findings of other similar studies.
   d. All of the above.
   e. None of the above; quasi-experimental studies cannot be generalized.

Activity 5: Evidence-Based Practice Activity

When using evidence-based practice strategies, the first step is to decide which level of evidence a research article provides. Review Figure 1-1 in the textbook, and determine the level of evidence (I, II, III, VI, or V) for each of the following.

1. A committee of neonatal experts at your local hospital issues an opinion paper.

2. An advanced-practice oncology nursing society conducted an evidence-based study of systematic reviews and issued a clinical practice guideline about catheter infection prevention.

3. A single phenomenological study examined the lived experience of being homeless and pregnant.

4. A large randomized controlled clinical trial is conducted.

5. A single study used a nonequivalent control group design.

POSTTEST

1. Identify whether the following studies are *experimental* (E) or *quasi-experimental* (Q).

   a. ________ Fifty teen mothers are randomly assigned to an experimental parenting support group and a regular support group. Before the program and at the end of the 3-month program, mother–child interaction patterns are compared between the two groups.

   b. ________ Patients on two separate units are given a patient satisfaction with care questionnaire to complete at the end of their first hospital day and on the day of discharge. The patients on one unit receive care directed by a nurse case manager, and the patients on the other unit receive care from the usual rotation of nurses. Patient satisfaction scores are compared.

   c. ________ Students are randomly assigned to two groups. One group receives an experimental independent study program and the other receives the usual classroom instruction. Both groups receive the same posttest to evaluate learning.

   d. ________ A study was conducted to compare the effectiveness of a music relaxation program with silent relaxation on lowering blood pressure ratings. Participants were randomly assigned into groups and blood pressures were measured before, during, and immediately after the relaxation exercises.

   e. ________ Reading and language development skills were compared between a group of children with chronic otitis media and a group of children without a history of ear problems.

2. Identify the type of experimental or quasi-experimental design for each of the following examples. Use the numbers from the key provided.

   Key: 1 = After-only
   2 = After-only nonequivalent control group
   3 = True experiment
   4 = Nonequivalent control group
   5 = Time series
   6 = Solomon four-group

   a. ________ Nurses are randomly assigned to a new self-study program or the usual electroencephalogram (EEG) teaching program. Knowledge of EEGs is tested before and after the program for both groups.

   b. ________ Babies who tested positive on toxicology screening at birth are randomly assigned to groups to receive either routine care or a special public health nurse intervention program. Health outcomes are tested and compared at 6 months.

   c. ________ A school nurse clinic is set up at one school. Health care outcomes are measured at the end of a year from that school and compared with health outcomes at a comparable school that does not have a clinic.

   d. ________ Diabetic patients were randomly assigned to either one of two control groups receiving routine home health care or to one of two groups with a new diabetic teaching program. Patients in one of the control groups and in one of the teaching groups took a test of diabetic knowledge as soon as they were assigned to a group. Patients in the other two groups were not pretested. All patients completed a posttest at the conclusion of the 3-week program.

   e. ________ A new peer AIDS prevention program was implemented in one high school. A second high school without the program served as a control group. An AIDS knowledge test was administered at both schools before and after the program was completed.

   f. ________ Trends in patient falls were summarized each week 1 year before and for the first year after implementation of a new hospital-based quality assurance program.

REFERENCES

Nyamathi, A., Salem, B., Zhang, S., Farabee, D., Hall, B., Khalilifard, F., & Leake, B. (2015). Nursing case management, peer coaching, and hepatitis A and B vaccine completion among homeless men recently released on parole: A randomized trial. *Nursing Research, 64*(3), 177-189.

10 Nonexperimental Designs

INTRODUCTION

Nonexperimental designs can provide extensive amounts of data that may help fill in the gaps found in nursing research. These designs help us clarify, see the real world, and assess relationships between variables, and they can provide clues that direct future, more controlled research. In this way, experimental, quasi-experimental, and nonexperimental designs complement each other. Each provides necessary components of our knowledge base. Nonexperimental designs allow us to discover some of the territory of nursing knowledge before trying to rearrange parts of it. It can be the base on which knowledge is built and further refined with quasi-experimental and experimental research.

LEARNING OUTCOMES

On completion of this chapter, you should be able to do the following:

- Describe the purpose of nonexperimental designs.
- Describe the characteristics of nonexperimental designs.
- Define the differences between nonexperimental designs.
- List the advantages and disadvantages of nonexperimental designs
- Identify the purpose and methods of methodological, secondary analysis, and mixed method designs.
- Identify the critical appraisal criteria used to critique nonexperimental research designs.
- Evaluate the strength and quality of evidence by nonexperimental designs.

Activity 1

Match the following definitions in Column A with the appropriate terms in Column B.

Column A

1. ________ This type is better known for the breadth than the depth of data collected.
2. ________ A major disadvantage is the length of time needed for data collection.
3. ________ The main question is whether or not variables covary.
4. ________ These words mean *after the fact.*
5. ________ This eliminates the confounding variable of maturation.
6. ________ This quantifies the magnitude and direction of a relationship.
7. ________ Collects data from the same group at several points in time.
8. ________ Can be surprisingly accurate if the sample is representative.
9. ________ Uses data from one point in time.
10. ________ This is based on two or more naturally occurring groups with different conditions of the presumed independent variable.

Column B

a. Comparative
b. Cross-sectional
c. Correlational
d. Ex post facto
e. Longitudinal
f. Survey

Activity 2

Following are a series of advantages and disadvantages for various types of nonexperimental designs. For each type of design, pick at least one *advantage* (A) and one *disadvantage* (D) from the list that accurately describes a quality of the design. Then insert the A or D with the appropriate number in the list below.

	Advantages	Disadvantages
Correlation studies	________________	________________
Cross-sectional	________________	________________
Ex post facto	________________	________________
Longitudinal	________________	________________
Prospective	________________	________________
Retrospective	________________	________________
Survey	________________	________________

Advantages

A1 A great deal of information can be economically obtained from a large population.

A2 Ability to assess changes in the variables of interest over time.

A3 Explores relationships between variables that are inherently not manipulable.

A4 Offers a higher level of control than a correlational study.

A5 They facilitate intelligent decision-making using objective criteria to guide the process.

A6 Each participant is followed separately and serves as his or her own control.

A7 Stronger than retrospective studies because of the degree of control on extraneous variables.

A8 Less time consuming, less expensive, and thus more manageable for the researcher.

Disadvantages

D1 The researcher is unable to draw a causal linkage between two variables.

D2 An alternative hypothesis could be the reason for the relationships.

D3 The researcher is unable to manipulate the variables of interest.

D4 The researcher is unable to determine a causal relationship between variables because of lack of manipulation, control, and randomization.

D5 The information obtained tends to be superficial.

D6 The researcher must know sampling techniques, questionnaire construction, interviewing, and data analysis.

D7 No randomization in sampling is possible because preexisting groups are studied.

D8 Internal validity threats such as testing and mortality are present.

D9 Participant loss to follow-up and attrition may lead to unintended sample bias that affects external validity and generalizability of findings.

Activity 3

Each of the following is a description of nonexperimental studies. For each example, determine the type of design used from the list provided. Not all designs are used as examples, and some will be used more than once.

C	Correlation studies	P	Prospective
CS	Cross-sectional	R	Retrospective
E	Ex post facto	SC	Survey comparative
L	Longitudinal	SD	Survey descriptive
M	Methodological	SE	Survey exploratory
MA	Meta-analysis		

Remember, some studies use more than one type of nonexperimental design.

1. A public health education nurse working with a senior center surveyed all residents to determine their priorities for health education classes and events.

   Type of design: ________

2. A study of children ages 2 to 18 years with diabetes collected data every year. Information collected included health surveys, glycated hemoglobin (HbA1c) levels, 24-hour diet recall, and measurements of height and weight. Children were assessed yearly and were included in the study up to the age of 18 years; data were collected for 10 consecutive years.

   Type of design: ________

3. A study of 200 low-income seniors, approximately half Caucasian and half African American, explored the relationship between hypertension, depression, self-esteem, and health-seeking behaviors. The data were collected on one occasion.

   Type of design: ________

4. A study examined the relationship of maternal dietary choices and infant birth weight. Medical records of 1000 postpartum women were examined to determine dietary choices and the relationship of a vegetarian or vegan diet with infant birth weight.

   Type of design: ________

5. The relationship between hypertension and social interaction in elderly adults living in isolated rural areas was explored.

   Type of design: ________

6. Forty-seven items were initially developed for the Haber and Wood Student Assessment Tool (HWSAT) after a thorough examination of the literature. These items were reviewed for relevance to the domain of content by a panel of eight experts using content validation.

   Type of design: ________

7. The purpose of this study was to examine the effect of simulation in nursing education and pass rates on board examinations. The LoBiondo-Wood Model of concept development was used in this study. An electronic search of the literature in several databases (CINAHL, MEDLINE, PubMed, Scopus) was conducted to find studies of the effectiveness of simulation on board exam pass rates in the nursing literature. The study used statistical analysis of 23 quantitative studies that met predetermined inclusion criteria to evaluate the effect of simulation on board pass rates.

   Type of design: ________

Activity 4

Use the critiquing criteria from the chapter to analyze the study by Turner-Sack et al. (2016) (see Appendix D in the textbook). In this study, the objective was to examine relationships of psychological functioning, posttraumatic growth, coping, and cancer-related characteristics of adolescent cancer survivors' parents and siblings.

1. What was the type of design?
   a. Longitudinal
   b. Cross-sectional
   c. Methodological
   d. Meta-analysis
   e. Correlational

2. Did the authors publish their hypotheses? If so, what were they?

3. What were the inclusion and exclusion criteria, and how do they relate to the study aims?

4. How often were data collected?

Activity 5

Review the Critical Thinking Decision Path: Nonexperimental Design Choice in the textbook. If you wanted to test a relationship between two variables in the past such as the incidence of reported back injuries of nurses working in newborn nurseries compared with those nurses working in long-term care, which design would you use?

Activity 6: Evidence-Based Practice Activity

1. What is the value of nonexperimental studies, such as ones that demonstrate a strong relationship in predictive correlational studies for evidence-based practice?
   a. They have no value.
   b. They provide evidence only for training purposes.
   c. They demonstrate cause-and-effect relationships and can be used in decision-making regarding changes in practice.
   d. They lend support for attempting to influence the independent variable in a future intervention study.

2. Which of the following nonexperimental designs provides a quality of evidence for evidence-based practice that is stronger than the others because the researcher can determine the incidence of a problem and its possible causes?
   a. Cross-sectional
   b. Longitudinal cohort
   c. Survey

3. When you, the research consumer, are using the evidence-based practice model to consider a change in practice, you will initially make your decision based on the strength and quality of evidence provided by the meta-analysis. After this, what other two characteristics will be important for you to consider? (There are two correct responses.)
   a. Clinical expertise
   b. Patient values
   c. Strength of the evidence
   d. Quality of the evidence
   e. Literature review

POSTTEST

Choose from among the following words to complete the posttest. Each word may be used one time; however, this list duplicates some words because they are used in more than one answer.

Comparative	Exploratory	Methodological	Retrospective
Correlational	Ex post facto	Prospective	Retrospective
Cross-sectional	Interrelational	Prospective	Survey
Cross-sectional	Longitudinal	Relationship- difference	Variables
Descriptive	Longitudinal	Retrospective	

1. In comparative surveys, the researcher does not manipulate the ____________________, but assesses data in order to provide evidence for future nursing intervention studies.
2. ____________________ is the broadest category of nonexperimental design.
3. The category from item 2 can be further classified as ____________________, ____________________, and ____________________.
4. The second major category of nonexperimental design, according to LoBiondo-Wood and Haber, includes ____________________ studies.
5. The researcher is using ____________________ design when examining the relationship between two or more variables.
6. ____________________ designs have many similarities to quasi-experimental designs.
7. ____________________ design used in epidemiological work is similar to ex post facto.
8. LoBiondo-Wood and Haber discuss three types of developmental studies. What are they?
   a. ____________________
   b. ____________________
   c. ____________________
9. ____________________ studies collect data at one point in time, whereas ____________________ collects data from the same group at different points in time.
10. A(n) ____________________ study looks at presumed causes and moves forward in time to presumed effects.
11. The researcher is using a(n) ____________________ design if he or she is trying to link present events to events that have occurred in the past.
12. The ____________________ researcher is interested in identifying an intangible construct (concept) and making it tangible with a paper-and-pencil instrument or observation protocol.

REFERENCES

Turner-Sack, A. M., Menna, R., Setchell, S. R., Maan, C., & Cataudella, D. (2016). Psychological functioning, post traumatic growth, and coping in parents and siblings of adolescent cancer survivors. *Oncology Nursing Forum, 43*(1), 48-56.

11 Systematic Reviews and Clinical Practice Guidelines

INTRODUCTION

Systematic reviews and clinical practice guidelines that assess multiple studies based on a single clinical question are an important element in many evidence-based practice problems. These studies provide an important means for organizing and analyzing the quality, consistency, and quantity of research findings. Thus it is important to have an understanding of the differences between the types of systematic reviews and clinical guidelines and to develop critiquing skills, so that when you find meaningful results for your clinical question, you can have a solid foundation for understanding the conduct and content of these studies.

LEARNING OUTCOMES

On completion of this chapter, you should be able to do the following:

- Describe the types of research reviews.
- Describe the components of a systematic review.
- Differentiate among a systematic review, a meta-analysis, and an integrative review.
- Describe the purpose of clinical guidelines.
- Differentiate between an expert-based and an evidence-based clinical guideline.
- Critically appraise systematic reviews and clinical practice guidelines.

Activity 1

Fill in the blanks for the following statements. Not all terms will be used and some terms may be used more than once.

Column A

1. A(n) ________________________ is a form of ________________________; however, the statistical analysis inherent in this type of study differentiates it from other broad categories of reviews. Clinical practice guidelines
2. A(n) ____________________ is the most general category of review and synthesizes the findings of quantitative or qualitative studies without using a statistical analysis.
3. A(n) ____________________ provides level I evidence.
4. Statements or recommendations that are systematically developed for clinicians are known as ________________________.
5. Whereas ____________________ are based on the opinions of experts in a field, ________________________ are developed using a scientific process.

Column B

Evidence-based guidelines
Expert-based guidelines
Integrative review
Meta-analysis
Randomized controlled trial (RCT)
Systematic review

Activity 2

Think about the components of a systematic review (you may also want to refer to Box 11-1) and decide which components add to or fulfill the following qualities of a high-quality systematic review. Use the following choices:

a. Clear aims
b. Transparency and reproducibility
c. Rigorous search
d. Validity assessment
e. Systematic presentation

1. ________ The authors fully describe their search strategy, provide evidence that all relevant databases were searched, and used these sources to comb through literature cited sections and bibliographies to use all possible sources for evidence.

2. ________ The aims are clearly stated as a population, intervention, comparison, outcome (PICO) statement. Eligibility and relevance criteria are well described and are predetermined. The reader can clearly see how the search relates to the aims and how studies included in the review fit eligibility criteria.

3. ________ The authors provide the reader with a way to identify the studies used in the review and their findings and quality. Often this is done in a table format. A good-quality table will allow the reader to understand the findings and will often lead naturally to a discussion where the author can easily synthesize the findings of the included studies.

4. ________ Readers should feel confident that based on the article, they could recreate the literature search, data extraction, bias assessment, data combination, and quality appraisal and reach the same conclusions as the authors. The authors should also fully describe their inclusion and exclusion criteria and the rationale behind them.

5. ________ The authors document how they determined validity and reliability of the studies in the review. (Did they use a quality appraisal system? If so, which one?) The authors provide their grading scheme for determination of quality in the included studies. The reader understands how the authors appraised the literature and how this appraisal led to the authors' conclusions in the paper. The experience and qualifications of all reviewers should also be briefly described.

Activity 3

All of the following statements are about systematic reviews and clinical guidelines. For each statement, determine the type(s) of reviews or guidelines described by the statement and write the abbreviation for each type in the box after the statement. Each statement may be described by more than one type of review or guideline.

SR: Systematic review
MA: Meta-analysis
IR: Integrative review
ECG: Expert-based clinical guideline
EBCG: Evidence-based clinical guideline

1. A summary of studies systematically found in the literature; focuses on a clearly stated question with a critical appraisal of the findings in a that area	
2. A method for searching and integrating the literature related to a specific clinical issue	
3. A review that uses statistical methods to assess and combine studies of the same design	
4. May review research literature, theoretical literature, or both; may include quantitative and/or qualitative research	

5. Statements or recommendations that link research and practice to guide practitioners	
6. Guidelines based on a rigorous literature search complete with an evidence table showing the quality and strength of the evidence on which the guideline is based	
7. Can provide a precise estimate of *effect*	
8. Guidelines for areas of clinical practice without a sufficient research base; often use expert opinion and whatever research is available	
9. Could be evaluated using the AGREE II instrument to determine quality and applicability to practice	
10. The broadest category of review	
11. The Cochrane Collaboration is a large repository of these	

Activity 4: Evidence-Based Practice Activity

1. What is the value of systematic reviews in evidence-based practice? List at least three.

2. You have a strong meta-analysis and other supporting literature on your clinical question. What else do you need to consider before you think about a change in clinical practice?

3. When you, the research consumer, are evaluating a meta-analysis to consider a change in practice, which two of the following characteristics are most important to consider when critiquing the evidence?
   a. Number of authors in the study
   b. Strength of the evidence
   c. Readability of the literature review
   d. Quality of the evidence
   e. Inclusion of patient preference in the study

4. Review Figure 1-1, Levels of evidence: Evidence hierarchy for rating levels of evidence, associated with a study's design, from your text.
   a. For each level of evidence in the left column, write in the center column the best description from the following list: systematic review of qualitative studies, well-designed RCT, single descriptive or qualitative study, meta-analysis of RCTs, quasiexperimental study, opinion of authorities, report of expert committee, single nonexperimental study.

b. For each level, indicate the source of evidence: A, expert opinion; B, qualitative; C, quantitative; D, combination of qualitative and quantitative; or E, anecdotal.

Level of Evidence	Description	Source
Level I		
Level II		
Level III		
Level IV		
Level V		
Level VI		
Level VII		

POSTTEST

Fill in the blanks to complete the posttest.

1. ______________________________ is the broadest category of review.

2. A systematic review is a summary of the ___________________ research literature on a focused clinical question.

3. The terms ___________________ and _____________________ are often used interchangeably, but after completing this chapter, I know that a(n) ___________________ uses statistical methods for the analysis of studies.

4. In a systematic review, it is important that _______________________ independently evaluates and critiques the studies included and _________________ in the review.

5. A(n) _________________________ provides the _________________________________ because it analyzes and integrates the results of many studies.

6. A meta-analysis and a systematic review include the same components, except for the ________________ of the studies.

7. It is important for a consumer of the literature to evaluate systematic reviews for potential ______________.

8. A(n) _____________________ is a graphic depiction of the results of a number of studies; it can also be called a(n) ________________________.

9. ________________________ guidelines are developed using a scientific process including a rigorous literature search, completion of an evidence table, and summary of the quality and strength of the evidence used to make each guideline. In areas without a sufficient research base, a group of experts can use their opinions and available research to develop ______________________.

10. Researchers who conduct a systematic review _________________ conduct the studies used in the review; rather, they use data from _________________ and synthesize the information following a set of systematic methods for combining evidence.

12 Sampling

INTRODUCTION

Sampling is a process of selection in which individuals, objects, animals, or events are chosen to represent the population of a study. The ideal sampling strategy is one in which the elements truly represent the population being studied while controlling for any source of bias. The specific research question determines the selection of the sample, variables to measure, and a sampling frame. The sampling strategies are important and should enable the choice of a sample that represents the target population and controls for bias as much as possible to ensure that the research will be valid. Reality modulates the ideal with the consideration of sampling in relation to efficiency, practicality, ethics, and availability of participants, which can alter the ideal strategy for a given study.

LEARNING OUTCOMES

On completion of this chapter, you should be able to do the following:

- Identify the purpose of sampling.
- Define *population, sample,* and *sampling.*
- Compare a population and a sample.
- Discuss the importance of inclusion and exclusion criteria.
- Define *nonprobability* and *probability sampling.*
- Identify the types of nonprobability and probability sampling strategies.
- Compare the advantages and disadvantages of specific nonprobability and probability sampling strategies.
- Discuss the contribution of nonprobability and probability sampling strategies to strength of evidence provided by study findings.
- Discuss the factors that influence sample size.
- Discuss potential threats to internal and external validity as sources of sampling bias.
- Use the critiquing criteria to evaluate the "Sample" section of a research report.

Activity 1

Write a short definition of each of the following and explain the differences between each set of words.

1. Sample: ______________________

   Population: ______________________

   Differences: ______________________

2. Target population: ______________________

   Accessible population: ______________________

   Differences: ______________________

3. Inclusion criteria: ______________________

   Exclusion criteria: ______________________

   Differences: ______________________

Activity 2

1. Is probability or nonprobability sampling more rigorous? Why?

2. Identify the category of sampling for each of the following sampling strategies. Use the abbreviations from the key provided.

Key:

P = Probability sampling
N = Nonprobability sampling

a. ________ Convenience sampling

b. ________ Purposive sampling

c. ________ Simple random sampling

d. ________ Quota sampling

e. ________ Cluster sampling

f. ________ Stratified random sampling

Activity 3

For each of the following examples of studies, identify the sampling strategy used from the following list. Write a letter that corresponds to the strategy in the space preceding the sampling description. Check the glossary for definition of terms. Strategies may be used more than once.

a. Convenience sampling
b. Quota sampling
c. Purposive sampling
d. Simple random sampling
e. Stratified random sampling

1. ________ The sample for the study of critical thinking behavior of undergraduate baccalaureate nursing students consisted of students enrolled in junior- and senior-level courses in three specific schools of nursing. In each program, students were invited to participate until a total sample representing 10% of the junior-level students and 10% of the senior-level students was obtained.

2. ________ Using a table of random numbers, the sample of 50 participants was selected from a list of all patients giving birth in the county during the first 6 months of the year.

3. ________ The sample was selected from residents of eight nursing homes in Arkansas and consisted of cognitively impaired people with no physical impairments or other psychiatric illness.

4. ________ The sample selected was parents who were chosen because of their knowledge and experience of having been a parent of a child in a neonatal intensive care unit (NICU). Inclusion criteria included those parents with a child admitted to the NICU for more than a week, gestation at birth 26 weeks or later, on a ventilator for at least 3 days, and discharged home within the last 6 months.

5. ________ The sample consisted of adolescent mothers, meeting eligibility requirements, who were recruited from referrals to the Community Health Services Division of the County Health Department until the sample reached a target number of 144 participants. Using a computer-based program, the patients were randomly assigned into one of two groups.

6. ________ To study the educational opportunities for nurses in various ethnic groups, a list of all nurses in the state of California was sorted by ethnicity. The sample consisted of 10% of the nurses in each ethnic group, selected according to a table of random numbers.

7. ________ A total of 155 infants were enrolled and divided into an intervention group of 72 infants and a control group of 83 infants. A computer program that generated random numbers assigned infants to intervention or control group.

Activity 4

1. Refer to the study by Hawthorne et al. (2016) in Appendix B of the textbook.

   a. Is the sample adequately described?

      Yes No

   b. Were there any differences between respondents and nonrespondents?

      Yes No Maybe

   c. What sampling strategy was used in this study?

   d. Is this a probability or nonprobability sample?

   e. What was the sampling unit?

      A. Place of death

      B. Family

      C. Individual

      D. Hospital

   f. What was the sample size?

2. List one advantage of using the sampling strategy described in this study.

3. List one disadvantage of using the sampling strategy described in this study.

Activity 5

Using the Critical Thinking Decision Path in the textbook, indicate whether the following statements are *true* (T) or *false* (F).

1. ________ Nonprobability sampling is associated with less generalizability to the larger population.
2. ________ Convenience sampling limits generalizability of findings largely because of the self-selection of participants.
3. ________ Nonprobability sampling strategies are more time consuming than probability strategies.
4. ________ Random sampling has the greatest risk of bias and is moderately representative.
5. ________ The easier the sampling strategy, the greater the risk of bias, and as sampling becomes easier to implement, the risk of bias and limited representativeness of the population increases.
6. ________ Purposive sampling procedures are the least generalizable sampling of the sampling strategies listed.
7. ________ Stratified random sampling uses a random selection procedure for obtaining sample participants.

Activity 6

Chapter 12 of the textbook provides an overview of sampling methods and introduces a variety of terms that have important implications for understanding research. Take some time to define the following terms in Column B and be sure that you can differentiate them, and then choose the best term to describe each of the following in Column A.

Column A

1. ________ A sampling strategy for a large national survey of public health nurses used a first sampling unit of states, then county, city, and department.
2. ________ The information collected about the most basic unit. In a study of neonates, this might be individuals or family units.
3. ________ A sample whose key characteristics closely match those of the population of interest.
4. ________ A research nurse selects a portion of all of the patients in a heart-transplant clinic to represent the entire population of the clinic.
5. ________ In a quantitative study of the lived experience of having an ileostomy, participants are added until no new data emerge during data collection.
6. ________ Researchers are trying to study a rare disease. They find an online network developed for people with the disease and ask the first participants they find to help them locate more participants meeting the eligibility criteria.
7. ________ A graduate student completes a small study using methods and procedures planned for use in a parent study. The study helps determine feasibility.
8. ________ Act as population descriptors; may include age, gender, socioeconomic status, level of education, religion, and ethnicity.
9. ________ In a study of students at Anytown High School each student in the school population has an equal and independent chance of being included in the sample.
10. ________ A research study makes measurements on these in the course of a study. They are the fundamental unit of the sample.
11. ________ In a study where the setting was all nursing schools in the United States, a list of all nursing schools in the nation would include all units of the population.

Column B

a. Element
b. Data saturation
c. Pilot study
d. Random selection
e. Sampling unit
f. Network (snowball) sampling
g. Multistage (cluster) sampling
h. Representative sample
i. Sampling frame
j. Delimitations
k. Sampling

Activity 7: Evidence-Based Practice Activity

The text defines *evidence-based practice* as the integration of best research evidence with clinical expertise and patient values. Evidence-based practice allows nurses to use research findings to make decisions to improve practice. Teams of nurses are applying multiple study findings to improve practice outcomes with individuals, families, and other health care professionals. Through this practice, more effective patient teaching and quality care are being realized.

What is the relationship between sampling and evidence-based practice decision-making? In other words, how will the sampling strategy in a study or a meta-analysis of studies influence how you and your colleagues make a decision about changing the practice in your health care setting? (Hint: Review the five Evidence-Based Practice Tips in Chapter 12 before answering this question.)

POSTTEST

Complete the following sentences.

1. A statistical technique known as __________________ may be used to determine sample size in quantitative studies.

2. Sampling strategies are grouped into two categories: __________________ sampling and __________________ sampling.

3. __________________ sampling is the use of the most readily accessible people or objects as participants in a study.

4. Advantages of __________________ sampling are low bias and maximal representativeness, but the disadvantage is the labor in drawing a sample.

5. A(n) __________________ can be used to select an unbiased sample or unbiased assignment of participants to treatment groups.

6. A(n) __________________ sample is one whose key characteristics closely approximate those of the population.

7. __________________ criteria are used to select the sample from all possible units and __________________ may be used to restrict the population to a homogeneous group of participants.

8. Types of nonprobability sampling include __________________, __________________, and __________________ sampling.

9. Successive random sampling of units that progress from large to small and meet sample eligibility criteria is known as __________________ sampling.

10. In certain qualitative studies, participants are added to the sample until __________________ occurs (new data no longer emerge during data collection).

REFERENCE

Hawthorne, D. M., Youngblut, J. M., & Brooten, D. (2016). Parent spirituality, grief, and mental health at 1 and 3 months after their infant's/child's death in an intensive care unit. *Journal of Pediatric Nursing, 31*(1), 73-80.

13 Legal and Ethical Issues

INTRODUCTION

Patient advocacy is one of the primary roles of a professional nurse. Nowhere is this more important than in the field of research. The nurse must be a patient advocate, whether acting as the researcher, a participant in data gathering, a provider of care for research participants, or a research consumer. A multitude of legal and ethical issues exist in research; nurses must be aware of, assess, act on, and evaluate these issues. In addition, nurses need to be knowledgeable about the purpose and functions of the institutional review board (IRB) and the federal regulations on which they are based.

LEARNING OUTCOMES

On completion of this chapter, you should be able to do the following:

- Describe the historical background that led to the development of ethical guidelines for the use of human participants in research.
- Identify the essential elements of an informed consent form.
- Evaluate the adequacy of an informed consent form.
- Describe the institutional review board's role in the research review process.
- Identify populations of participants who require special legal and ethical research considerations.
- Describe the nurse's role as patient advocate in research situations.
- Critique the ethical aspects of a research study.

Activity 1

Fill in the blanks in Column A with the correct term from Column B (not all of the terms will be used).

Column A

1. _____ __________________ reviews proposals for scientific merit and congruence with the institutional policies and missions.
2. _____ __________________ reviews research proposals to ensure protection of the rights of human participants.
3. _____ The idea that human participants should be treated fairly and should not be denied a benefit to which the participant is entitled is __________________.
4. _____ A study of existing data that is of minimal risk to participants may be a candidate for a(n) __________________.
5. _____ The U.S. Public Health Service studied the effects of untreated syphilis on African-American sharecroppers in Tuskegee, Alabama, and withheld penicillin treatment even after penicillin was commonly available. This is considered a(n) __________________.
6. _____ The regulation that requires the health care profession to protect the privacy of patient information and create standards for electronic data exchange is known as __________________.

Column B

a. Beneficence
b. Justice
c. Confidentiality
d. Nursing research committee
e. Expedited review
f. Unauthorized research
g. Institutional review board
h. Unethical research study
i. HIPAA
j. Respect for person

Activity 2

List the three ethical principles relevant to the conduct of research involving human participants. These were included in the Belmont Report (1979) and formed the basis for regulations affecting research sponsored by the federal government.

a. Beneficence
b. Justice
c. Confidentiality
d. Nursing research committee
e. Expedited review
f. Unauthorized research
g. Institutional review board
h. Unethical research study
i. HIPAA
j. Respect for person

1. ______________________________

2. ______________________________

3. ______________________________

Activity 3

Read the following example of a research consent form. Then review the list of the elements of informed consent that follows the example. For each item in the list of elements of informed consent, put either a "√" if the element is included in the consent or a "0" if it is absent from the consent. Summarize your findings in a paragraph at the end of the exercise.

Research Consent Form

Agreement to Participate in Research

Responsible Investigator: Mary Jo Gorney-Moreno, PhD, Professor, Nursing

Title of Protocol: A web-based interactive program to engage nurses in learning principles of pain management

We are recruiting nursing students to test a web-based interactive program to engage nurses in learning principles of pain management. There are three learning outcomes for this program: to (1) teach appropriate and safe control of the patient's pain, (2) teach prevention and management of side effects of pain management, and (3) provide accurate and complete patient teaching regarding pain and side effect management. At the end of the simulation, you will receive three scores, one for how well you managed patient care in each of these areas. It will take about 30 minutes to complete the simulation. The simulation is available online at http://www.cdl.edu/painless. You can complete the simulation as many times as you like; each time you will be presented with a new set of variables for the patient, Mr. Sanchez. The variables are programmed to appear randomly. We hope that this activity will enhance your knowledge related to providing pain management for your patients. There are no known risks for participation.

If you agree to participate, we welcome you and would like you to complete a pre- and posttest, as well as a short evaluation form after you complete the simulation. Your participation is voluntary, and you may withdraw at any time and for any reason. There is no penalty for not participating or withdrawing. The personal benefits for participation include assisting faculty and yourself to understand more about the effectiveness of this innovative educational intervention and to increase your knowledge. There are no costs to you or any other party.

I will ask you to print a copy of your scores from the simulation and complete the pre- and posttest and a short questionnaire. All data collected will be coded using a unique five-character string and will not be identified with you personally. There is no risk to you.

Dr. Mary Jo Gorney-Moreno, Professor, School of Nursing, San Jose State University, is conducting this study. Dr. Gorney-Moreno can be reached at 408-555-1000. You should understand that your participation is voluntary and that choosing not to participate in this study, or in any part of this study, will not affect your relations with San Jose State University. You may refuse to participate in the entire study or in any part of the study; you are free to withdraw at any time without any negative effect on your relations with San Jose State University. The results of this study may be published, but any information that could result in your identification will remain confidential. If you have questions about this study, I will be happy to talk with you. I can be reached at (408)-555-1020. If you have questions or complaints about research participants' rights, or in the event of a research-related injury, please contact Serena Smith, PhD, Associate Vice President for Graduate Studies and Research, at (408) 555-1040.

This project has been reviewed and approved according to the San Jose State University Human Subjects Institutional Review Board procedures governing human participants research.

Your signature indicates that you have been fully informed of your rights and voluntarily agree to participate in this study. You will be given a copy of this signed form.

By signing this form, I agree to participate in this study.

________________________ ________________________

Participant's Signature Date

Elements of Informed Consent

1. _______ Title of protocol
2. _______ Invitation to participate
3. _______ Basis for participant selection
4. _______ Overall purpose of the study
5. _______ Explanation of benefits
6. _______ Description of risks and discomforts
7. _______ Potential benefits
8. _______ Alternatives to participation
9. _______ Financial obligations
10. _______ Assurance of confidentiality
11. _______ In case of injury compensation
12. _______ HIPAA disclosure
13. _______ Participant withdrawal
14. _______ Offer to answer questions
15. _______ Concluding consent statement
16. _______ Identification of investigators

Activity 4

Nurses must be aware of populations that require special legal and ethical considerations. List at least four groups of participants who are vulnerable or have diminished autonomy and thus require extra protection as research participants.

1. ______________________________

2. ______________________________

3. ______________________________

4. ______________________________

Activity 5

Match the violation of ethical principles described in the following list with the examples presented below. More than one violation may have occurred in the examples that are cited. List all that were violated.

a. Degree of risk outweighed benefits
b. Participants not informed they could withdraw from study at any time
c. Participants not informed or offered the effective treatment that was available
d. Lack of informed consent
e. No evidence of IRB approval before start of research
f. Right to fair treatment and protection
g. Principles of informed consent violated or incomplete disclosure of potential risk, harm, results, or side effects given

1. Write the letter(s) describing violation after the description of the study.

   The UCLA Schizophrenic Medication Study was a 1983 study examining the effects of withdrawing psychotropic medications on 50 patients under treatment for schizophrenia. Twenty-three participants suffered severe relapses after their medications were stopped. The goal of the study was to determine if some schizophrenics might do better without medications that had deleterious side effects. Patients were not informed that their symptoms could worsen or about the severity of a potential relapse. ________________

2. List the letter(s) that correspond(s) to the ethical violation(s) described.

   The United States Public Health Service conducted a study from 1932 to 1973 on two groups of poor male African-American sharecroppers. One group had untreated syphilis and the other did not. Treatment was withheld from the group diagnosed with syphilis, even after it became generally available and was known to be effective. Steps were taken to prevent infected participants from obtaining penicillin. The researchers wanted to study the effects of untreated syphilis. ________________

Activity 6

This activity assesses the use of procedures for protecting basic human rights. Review the articles in Appendices A through D of the text. For each article, describe how informed consent was obtained, and determine whether the author described obtaining permission from the institutional review board.

1. Nyamathi et al. (2015): ______________________________

____

____

2. Hawthorne et al. (2016): ______________________________

____

____

3. van Dijk (2016): ______________________________

____

____

4. Turner-Sack et al. (2016): ______________________________

____

____

Activity 7: Evidence-Based Practice Activity

You are a nurse working in a postpartum unit. If you decided to make a change in your practice based on an evidence-based practice article, but first wanted to check to be certain that no misconduct had occurred in the conduct or reporting of the study, where would you find this information?

POSTTEST

1. It is necessary for researchers and nurses to protect the basic human rights of vulnerable groups. Can research studies be conducted with these populations?

   Yes, because ______________________________

   No, because ______________________________

2. A researcher must receive IRB approval (before/after) beginning to conduct research involving humans.

3. If you question whether a researcher has permission to conduct a study in your hospital, which documents would you want to see that demonstrate approval from which group(s)? ______________________________

____

4. Should a researcher list all the possible risks and benefits of participating in a research study even if some people may refuse because these items are listed in detail?

   Yes No

5. If you agreed to collect data for a researcher who had not asked the patient's permission to participate in the research study, you would be violating the patient's right to ________________.

6. What are two of the risks of scientific fraud or misconduct? ____

   ____

REFERENCES

Hawthorne, D. M., Youngblut, J. M., & Brooten, D. (2016). Parent spirituality, grief, and mental health at 1 and 3 months after their infant's/child's death in an intensive care unit. *Journal of Pediatric Nursing, 31*(1), 73-80.

Nyamathi, A., Salem, B. E., Zhang, S., Farabee, D., Hall, B., Khalilifard, F., & Leake, B. (2015). Nursing care management, peer coaching, and hepatitis A and B vaccine completion among homeless men recently released on parole. *Nursing Research, 64*(3), 177-189.

Turner-Sack, A. M., Menna, R., Setchell, S. R., Maan, C., & Cataudella, D. (2016). Psychological functioning, post traumatic growth, and coping in parents and siblings of adolescent cancer survivors. *Oncology Nursing Forum, 43*(1), 48-56.

van Dijk, J. F. M., Vervoort, S. C. J. M., van Wijck, A. J. M., Kalkman, C. J., & Schuurmans, M. J. (2016). Postoperative patients' perspective on rating pain: A qualitative study. *International Journal of Nursing Studies, 53,* 260-269.

14 Data Collection Methods

INTRODUCTION

Observe, probe
Details unfold
Let nature's secrets
Be stammeringly retold.

—Goethe

The focus of this chapter is basic information about data collection. As a consumer of research, the reader needs the skills to evaluate and critique data collection methods in published research studies. To achieve these skills, it is helpful to have an appreciation of the process or the critical thinking "journey" the researcher has taken to be ready to collect the data. Each of the preceding chapters represented important preliminary steps in the research planning and designing phases before data collection. Although most researchers are eager to begin data collection, the planning for data collection is very important. The planning includes identifying and prioritizing data needs, developing or selecting appropriate data collection tools, and selecting and training data collection personnel before proceeding with actual collection of data.

The five types of data collection methods differ in their basic approach and in the strengths and weaknesses of their characteristics. Readers should be prepared to ask questions about the appropriateness of the measures chosen by the researcher to gather data about the variable of concern. This includes determining the objectivity, consistency, quantifiability, observer intervention, and obtrusiveness of the chosen data collection method.

LEARNING OUTCOMES

On completion of this chapter, you should be able to do the following:

- Define the types of data collection methods used in nursing research.
- List the advantages and disadvantages of each data collection method.
- Compare how specific data collection methods contribute to the strength of evidence in a research study.
- Identify potential sources of bias related to data collection.
- Discuss the importance of intervention fidelity in data collection.
- Critically evaluate the data collection methods used in published research studies.

Activity 1

Review each of the following referenced articles. Be especially thorough in reading the sections that relate to data collection methods. Answer the questions in relation to what you understand from the article. For some questions, there may be more than one answer.

Study 1

Nyamathi et al., 2016 (in Appendix A of the textbook).

1. Which data collection method(s) is/are used in this research study?
   a. A physiological measure
   b. An observational measure
   c. An interview measure
   d. A questionnaire measure
   e. Records of available data

2. In your opinion, what would be the advantage in using this (these) method(s)? What explanation do the investigators provide?

Study 2

Hawthorne et al., 2016 (in Appendix B of the textbook)

1. Which data collection method is used in this research study?
   a. A physiological measure
   b. An observational measure
   c. An interview measure
   d. A questionnaire
   e. Records of available data

2. What is the rationale for the appropriateness of the data collection method(s)?

Study 3

Van Dijk et al., 2016 (in Appendix C of the textbook)

1. What data collection method is used in this research study?
   a. A physiological measure
   b. An observational measure
   c. An interview measure
   d. A questionnaire
   e. Records of available data

2. What were the strengths and weaknesses of using this method?

Study 4

Turner-Sack et al., 2016 (in Appendix D of the textbook)

1. What data collection method is used in this research study?
   a. A physiological measure
   b. An observational measure
   c. An interview measure
   d. A questionnaire
   e. Records of available data

2. Describe the data collection method.

3. What are two possible problems with self-report methods that might have affected the results in this study?

Activity 2

Using the content of Chapter 14 in the textbook, answer the questions in Column A using the terms in Column B. Not all answers will be used and some may be used more than once.

Column A

1. Baccalaureate-prepared nurses are ___________________ of research.
2. ___________________ methods use technical instruments to collect data about patients' physical, chemical, microbiological, or anatomical status.
3. ___________________ is the distortion of data as a result of the observer's presence.
4. ___________________ are best used when a large response rate and an unbiased sample are important.
5. ___________________ data collection method is subject to problems of availability, authenticity, and accuracy.
6. ___________________ measurements are especially useful when there are a finite number of questions to be asked and the questions are clear and specific.
7. Essential in the critique of data collection methods is the emphasis on the appropriateness, ___________________, and ___________________ of the method employed.
8. ___________________ raises ethical questions (especially informed consent issues); therefore, it is not often used in nursing.
9. ___________________ ___________________ is a common observational technique where the researcher functions as part of a social group in order to study the group in question.
10. ___________________ is the process of translating concepts and variables into measurable phenomena.
11. ___________________ is a format that uses closed-ended items, and there are a fixed number of alternative responses.
12. ___________________ is the method for objective, systematic, and quantitative description of communications and documentary evidence.

Column B

a. Anecdotes
b. Consumers
c. Concealment
d. Consistency
e. Content analysis
f. Interviews
g. Likert scales
h. Objectivity
i. Operationalization
j. Questionnaires
k. Participant observation
l. Physiological
m. Reactivity
n. Records
o. Respondent burden
p. Scale

Activity 3

You are reviewing a study, and concealment is necessary; in other words, there is no other way to collect the data, and the data collected will not have negative consequences for the participant.

1. Name at least one population where concealment is not uncommon.

2. How would you obtain participants' consent?

3. What is the major reason for using concealment?

Activity 4

Using the content of Chapter 14 in the textbook, circle the correct response for each question. Some questions will have more than one answer.

1. What is a primary advantage of physiological measures?
   a. The measuring tool never affects the phenomena being measured.
   b. It is one of the easiest types of methods to implement.
   c. It is unlikely that study participants can distort the physiological information.
   d. They offer objectivity, sensitivity, and precision.
   e. All of the above.

2. Self-report measures are usually more useful than observation measures in obtaining information about which of the following?
   a. Socially unacceptable or private behaviors
   b. Complex research situations when it is difficult to separate processes and interactions
   c. When the researcher is interested in character traits
   d. All of the above

3. Which of the following would be considered disadvantages of using observational data collection methods?
   a. Individual bias may interfere with the data collection.
   b. Ethical concerns may be increasingly significant to researchers using observational data collection methods.
   c. Individual judgments and values influence the perceptions of the observers.
   d. All of the above.

4. In nursing research, when might questionnaires be used as an appropriate method for data collection?
   a. Whenever expense is a concern for the researcher
   b. When a researcher is interested in obtaining information directly from the participants
   c. When the researcher needs to collect data from a large group of participants who are not easily accessible
   d. When accuracy is of the utmost importance to the researcher

5. Which of the following would be considered advantages of using existing records or available data to answer a research question?
   a. The use of available data reduces the risk of researcher bias in data collection.
   b. Time involvement in the research study can be reduced by the use of available records or data.
   c. Consistent collection of information over time allows the researcher to study trends.
   d. All of the above.

Activity 5: Evidence-Based Practice Activity

Check the evidence-based practice resources available at your clinical site or go to your library home page. Find the Cochrane Library or any database with access to evidence-based resources. Search for "nursing intervention." Choose a recent study of a nursing intervention you might use in your practice.

1. What were some of the methods used in studies included in this review? Were the methods appropriate?

2. Would you change your practice based on the evidence provided in this study? Explain your answer.

3. After looking at the Results and Discussion sections of the article you reviewed, how would you improve the data collection methods of the studies under review to strengthen the evidence?

POSTTEST

Read each question thoroughly and then circle the correct answer.

1. What is the process of translating concepts that are of interest to the researcher into observable and measurable phenomena?
   a. Objectivism
   b. Systematization
   c. Subjectivism
   d. Operationalization

2. Answering research questions pertaining to psychosocial variables can best be done by using which data-gathering technique(s)?
   a. Observation
   b. Interviews
   c. Questionnaires
   d. All of the above

3. Collection of data from each participant in the same or in a similar manner is known as
   a. repetition.
   b. dualism.
   c. consistency.
   d. recidivism.

4. Consistency of observations between two or more observers is known as
   a. intrarater reliability.
   b. interrater reliability.
   c. consistency reliability.
   d. repetitive reliability.

5. Physiological and biological measurement might be used by nurse researchers when studying which of these variables? (Select all that apply.)
   a. A comparison of student nurses' ACT scores and their GPAs
   b. Hypertensive clients' responses to a stress test
   c. Children's dietary patterns
   d. The degree of pain relief achieved after guided imagery

6. Scientific observations should fulfill which of the following conditions?
   a. Observations are consistent with the study objectives.
   b. Observations are standardized and systematically recorded.
   c. Observations are checked and controlled.
   d. All of the above.

7. In a research study, a participant observer spent regularly scheduled hours in a homeless shelter and occasionally stayed overnight. The people staying in the home were told that this person was conducting a research study. The researcher freely engaged in conversation and openly observed the homeless. What is the observational role of the researcher?
   a. Concealment without intervention
   b. Concealment with intervention
   c. No concealment without intervention
   d. No concealment with intervention

8. In unstructured observation, which of the following might occur? (Select all that apply.)
   a. Extensive field notes are recorded.
   b. Participants are informed what behaviors are being observed.
   c. The researcher frequently records interesting anecdotes.
   d. All of the above.

9. Which of the following is *not* consistent with a Likert scale?
   a. It contains closed-ended items.
   b. It contains open-ended items.
   c. It contains lists of statements.
   d. Items are evaluated on the amount of agreement.

10. Although it is acceptable to use multiple instruments within a research study, the study is more acceptable if only one method is used for the data collection.
   a. True
   b. False

11. Social desirability is seldom a concern for researchers when the data collection method used in the study is interviews.
   a. True
   b. False

12. A researcher desires to use a questionnaire in a study but cannot find one that will gather the information desired about a particular variable. The decision is made to develop a new instrument. Which of the following should the researcher do?
   a. Define the construct, formulate the items, and assess the items for content validity
   b. Develop instructions for users and pilot the instrument
   c. Estimate reliability and validity
   d. All of the above

13. The researcher who invests significant amounts of time in the development of an instrument has a professional responsibility to publish the results.
   a. True
   b. False

14. To evaluate the adequacy of various data collection methods, which of the following should be included in the written research report?
   a. Clear identification of the rationale for selecting a physiological measure is provided.
   b. The problems of bias and reactivity are addressed with observational measures.
   c. There is a clear explanation of how interviews were conducted and how interviewers were trained.
   d. All of the above.

15. In conducting a research study, the researcher has a responsibility to ensure that all study participants received the same information and data were collected from all participants in the same manner.
   a. True
   b. False

REFERENCES

Hawthorne, D. M., Youngblut, J. M., & Brooten, D. (2016). Parent spirituality, grief, and mental health at 1 and 3 months after their infant's/child's death in an intensive care unit. *Journal of Pediatric Nursing, 31*(1), 73-80.

Nyamathi, A., Salem, B. E., Zhang, S., Farabee, D., Hall, B., Khalilifard, F., & Leake, B. (2016). Nursing care management, peer coaching, and hepatitis A and B vaccine completion among homeless men recently released on parole. *Nursing Research, 64*(3), 177-189.

Turner-Sack, A. M., Menna, R., Setchell, S. R., Maan, C., & Cataudella, D. (2016). Psychological functioning, post traumatic growth, and coping in parents and siblings of adolescent cancer survivors. *Oncology Nursing Forum, 43*(1), 48-56.

van Dijk, J. F. M., Vervoort, S. C. J. M., van Wijck, A. J. M., Kalkman, C. J., & Schuurmans, M. J. (2016). Postoperative patients' perspective on rating pain: A qualitative study. *International Journal of Nursing Studies, 53,* 260-269.

15 Reliability and Validity

INTRODUCTION

If a friend tells you, "Hey, I found a new restaurant that you will really love," you will consider that information from at least two perspectives before you spend your money there. First, does this person understand your taste in food? Second, has this person given you good information about food in the past?

You answer "no" to the first question. You prefer seafood served in an elegant setting, and your friend prefers pizza served in a place with sawdust on the floor. Using this information, you will consider your friend's opinion to be invalid for you. You will never give this restaurant another thought.

But if you answer "yes" to the first question because you share similar tastes in food, you will move on to the second question. You remember the tough fettuccini, the superb Southern fried chicken, the unbaked pizza dough, and the hockey-puck biscuits from earlier recommendations. It is likely that although you and your friend share food preferences, her information is not reliable. You can't trust her to give you good information over time. If you are feeling like an adventure, you may try the new restaurant or you may not.

Validity and reliability of the data collection instruments used in a study are to be regarded in the same way that you would consider your friend's advice about restaurants. Is the instrument valid? Does it provide me with accurate information? Is the instrument reliable? Does it provide me with consistent information whenever it is used? Consideration of both validity and reliability influences your confidence in the results of the study.

LEARNING OUTCOMES

On completion of this chapter, you should be able to do the following:

- Discuss how measurement error can affect the outcomes of a research study.
- Discuss the purposes of reliability and validity.
- Define *reliability.*
- Discuss the concepts of stability, equivalence, and homogeneity as they relate to reliability.
- Compare and contrast the estimates of reliability.
- Define *validity.*
- Compare and contrast content, criterion-related, and construct validity.
- Identify the criteria for critiquing the reliability and validity of measurement tools.
- Use the critiquing criteria to evaluate the reliability and validity of measurement tools.
- Discuss how evidence related to reliability and validity contributes to the strength and quality of evidence provided by the findings of a research study.

Activity 1

Either random error (*R*) or systematic error (*S*) may occur in a research study. For each of the following examples, identify the type of measurement error and how the error might be corrected.

1. ________ The scale used to obtain daily weights was inaccurate by 3 pounds less than actual weight.

   Correction: ____

2. ________ Students chose the socially acceptable responses on an instrument to assess attitudes toward AIDS patients.

   Correction: ____

3. ________ Confusion existed among the evaluators on how to score the wound healing.

   Correction: ____

4. _______ The participants were nervous about taking the psychological tests.

Correction: ____

Activity 2

Validity is the extent to which a measurement tool actually measures the concepts it is supposed to measure. Use the terms from Column B to complete each of the items in Column A. (Not all terms will be used and some terms may be used more than once.)

Column A

1. _____ ________________ of the instrument was evaluated by exploratory factor analysis (EFA) and confirmatory factor analysis (CFA). Samples sizes for EFA and CFA were 632 and 578, respectively.

2. _____ ________________ is a rudimentary type of validity testing in which colleagues, experts, or participants read the instrument to evaluate if it reflects the concept the researcher is trying to measure.

3. _____ "________________ of the SCS subscales is supported by correlations of .40 with the well-established Spiritual Well Being Instrument." (Hawthorne et al., 2016)

4. _____ The authors and six doctoral students developed a one-page questionnaire titled "Travel Health." Occupational health nurses (n = 10) with graduate-level training and experience in travel health rated the scale's items for relevance to the construct and a ________________ was calculated using the average of the responses from the experts.

5. _____ The current study showed that when the Fatigue Symptom Scale and the TIRED Scale were given to the same participants and a correlational analysis was performed, there was ________________ based on the positive correlation between both measures of the concept of fatigue.

6. _____, _____, _____ Construct validity, an assessment of the relationship between the instrument and the underlying theory, can be measured in several ways. List three of these: ________________, ________________, and ________________.

7. _____ An instrument is being developed to measure physical activity in knee injury patients. The instrument was administered to a group of patients the day before surgery and another group of patients 6 months after surgery. A t test found significant differences between the groups. This is a ________________ test of construct validity.

Column B

a. Construct validity
b. Content validity index
c. Contrasted groups
d. Convergent validity
e. Criterion-related validity
f. Divergent validity
g. Face validity
h. Factor analysis
i. Hypothesis testing
j. Multitrait-multimethod approach
k. Predictive validity

Activity 3

An instrument is considered reliable if it is accurate and consistent. If the concept being studied is stable, the same results should occur when measurement is repeated. Use the following items to answer questions 1 and 2.

a. Alternate forms
b. Construct
c. Equivalence
d. Homogeneity
e. Kappa
f. Parallel forms
g. Stability
h. Test-retest

1. Three concepts related to reliability include __________________, __________________, and __________________.

2. What are two types of tests for stability? ______ and _______ Provide an example of each.

3. In what instance would it be better to use an alternate form rather than a test-retest measure for stability?

4. Homogeneity is a measure of internal consistency. All items on the instrument should be complementary and measure the same characteristic or concepts. For each of the following examples, identify which of the following tests for homogeneity is described:
   1. Item-total correlations
   2. Split-half reliability
   3. Kuder-Richardson (KR-20) coefficient
   4. Cronbach's alpha

   a. ________ The odd items of the test had a high correlation with the even numbers of the test.
   b. ________ Each item on the test using a five-point Likert scale had a moderate correlation with every other item on the test.
   c. ________ Each item on the test ranged in correlation from 0.62 to 0.89 with the total.
   d. ________ Each item on the true-false test had a moderate correlation with every other item on the test.

5. Review the following information about one of the instruments used in the study in Appendix D of the text and answer the questions below: "Life satisfaction: Survivors and siblings completed the Student's Life Satisfaction Scale (SLSS) (Heubner, 1991), a self-report questionnaire that assesses global life satisfaction in children and adolescents. Participants used a six-point scale ranging from 1 (strongly disagree) to 6 (strongly agree) to respond to seven statements about their lives. The average score per SLSS item was used in the analyses, with high scores indicating more life satisfaction. The internal consistency in the current study was 0.87 for survivors and siblings."

   "Coping strategies: The COPE (Carver, Scheier, & Weintraub, 1989) assesses coping strategies in adolescents and adults. Participants used this 60-item self-report questionnaire to rate the way they respond to stressful events. Participants used a four-point scale ranging from 1-4, with 1 indicating 'I usually do not do this at all,' and 4 indicating 'usually do this a lot.' The COPE yields scores on 15 different scales. Factor analyses have revealed slightly different factor structures for adolescents and adults. Phelps and Jarvis (1994) proposed a four-factor structure for adolescents: active coping, emotion-focused coping, avoidant coping, and acceptance coping. Similarly, Carver et al. (1989) proposed a four-factor structure for adults: active coping, social support and emotion-focused coping, avoidant coping, and acceptance coping. The current study used the four factors proposed by Phelps and Jarvis (1994) for the survivors and siblings and the four factors proposed by Carver et al. (1989) for the parents. The religious coping scale was not associated with any of the factors but was included for all groups. High scores on a particular factor or scale reflect a greater use of that type of coping strategy; in the current study, internal consistency ranged from 0.74 (acceptance coping) to 0.94 (religious coping) for survivors and siblings, and from 0.52 (avoidant coping) to 0.94 (religious coping) for parents." (Turner-Sack et al., 2016)

1. Parallel form
2. Likert scale
3. Item to total correlation
4. KR-20
5. Cronbach's alpha
6. Reliability
7. Validity
8. A value greater than .50
9. A value greater than .70
10. A value greater than .95

a. How would you describe the questions on the SLSS? ______

b. Based on what you know about SLSS and COPE type of instruments, what type of internal consistency measure is most likely?

c. When the authors state that "internal consistency ranged from 0.74 (acceptance coping) to 0.94 (religious coping) for survivors and siblings, and from 0.52 (avoidant coping) to 0.94 (religious coping) for parents," these numbers represent _______ of the study.

d. What numerical value would represent sufficient evidence for supporting the internal consistency of the instrument?

Activity 4

In this activity, you will use the critiquing criteria listed in Chapter 15 of the text to think about the Hawthorne et al. study in Appendix B of the text.

1. How many instruments for data collection were used in this study?

2. For the Beck Depression Inventory (BDI-II):

Answer questions a-g using the following terms. If prompted, please explain your answer. Choose from the following responses:

1. No
2. Yes
3. Cronbach's alpha
4. Test-retest reliability
5. Item-total correlation
6. Interitem correlation
7. Split half
8. Parallel or alternate form

a. What information on validity was included in the article?

b. Did the authors report on any tests of reliability?

c. Name some appropriate tests of reliability for this instrument.

d. Would a KR-20 test be a good test of reliability? Why or why not?

e. Has this instrument been previously used in this population?

f. If you wanted information on validity, where would you look?

g. Where in the article would you look to see how the results of this study compared with BDI-II scores from other studies?

Activity 5: Evidence-Based Practice Activity

Now think about the Turner-Sack et al. (2016) study. Look at the reliability and validity measures of the instruments used in the study. Assume you are a nurse who cares for adolescent cancer patients. How would you use the results of this study to guide your practice?

POSTTEST

Using the terms in Column B, complete the sentences in Column A for the type of validity or reliability discussed. (Terms may be used more than once.)

Column A

1. _____ In tests for reliability, the self-efficacy scale had a(n) ____________________ of 0.88, demonstrating internal consistency for the new measure.
2. _____ The ABC social support scale demonstrated ____________________ validity with correlation of 0.84 with the XYZ interpersonal relationships scale.
3. _____ ____________________ validity was supported with a correlation of 0.42 between the ABC social support scale and the QRS loneliness scale.
4. _____ The investigator established ____________________ validity through evaluation of the cardiac recovery scale by a panel of cardiac clinical nurse specialists. All items were rated 0 to 5 for importance to recovery and only items scoring above an average of 3 were kept in the final scale.
5. _____ The results of the ____________________ were that all the items clustered around three factors, lending support to the notion that there are three dimensions of coping.
6. _____ The observations were rated by three experts. The ____________________ reliability among the observers was 94%.
7. _____ To assess ____________________ reliability, participants completed the locus of control questionnaire at the beginning of the project and 2 weeks later. The correlation of 0.86 supports the stability of the concept.
8. _____ The Heart Health and Recovery Test (HHRT) was developed by the interdisciplinary heart health group. They established ____________________ validity by examining the literature reviewing concerns identified by patients recovering from a cardiac event and had the items critiqued by a panel of experts.
9. _____ The results of the HHRT that measured threat were highly correlated with the results of a test measuring negative emotions. This established ____________________ validity.
10. _____ The interdisciplinary heart health study group reported that internal consistency reliabilities of the five factors of the HHRT were computed with the ____________________ statistic.

Column B

a. Content
b. Factor analysis
c. Convergent
d. Divergent
e. Test-retest
f. Cronbach's alpha
g. Alternate or parallel form
h. Interrater
i. Concurrent

REFERENCES

Hawthorne, D. M., Youngblut, J. M., & Brooten, D. (2016). Parent spirituality, grief, and mental health at 1 and 3 months after their infant's/child's death in an intensive care unit. *Journal of Pediatric Nursing, 31*(1), 73-80.

Turner-Sack, A. M., Menna, R., Setchell, S. R., Maan, C., & Cataudella, D. (2016). Psychological functioning, post traumatic growth, and coping in parents and siblings of adolescent cancer survivors. *Oncology Nursing Forum, 43*(1), 48-56.

16 Data Analysis: Descriptive and Inferential Statistics

INTRODUCTION

Measurement is critical to any study. The practitioner is interested in the similarity between the measurements used in a study and those usually found in his or her practice. The researcher thinks about how to measure relevant variables while reading the literature and thinking through the theoretical rationale for the study. Both the practitioner and the researcher wonder about how much faith they can put in the measurements reported.

Practitioners and researchers know that the perfect set of measurements does not exist. The researcher's task is to clearly define the variables, choose accurate measurement tools, and clearly explain how the statistical tools were used. Your task as a practitioner who critically reads research is to consider the researcher's explanation of how and why specific descriptive and inferential statistics were used and ask, "What do these numbers tell me?"

Descriptive statistics are valuable for summarizing data and allowing us to look at salient features about a group of data, but practitioners usually want more information. They want to be able to read about an intervention used with a specific group of individuals and consider the usefulness of that intervention with the patients in their care. The use of inferential statistics provides a way for practitioners to look at the data in a study and decide how easily the results can be generalized to the patients they see on a daily basis.

Initially, numbers tend to be intimidating. The best way to eliminate this source of intimidation is to jump in and play with the numbers. Keep reminding yourself that you have the intelligence and skills to do this. Use the mantras of "I think I can. I think I can," and "Practice, practice, practice," and you will have data analysis mastered. Also keep in mind that this is a lifelong learning process. There will still be times when you read a study with a new twist to the use of a statistical procedure, and back you'll go to the reference books, or you'll pick up the phone to call a colleague.

This chapter is designed to help you with the skills part of the task. First, the exercises in this chapter will provide you with some practice in working with the concept of measurement. Second, you will have the opportunity to think through some of the decisions relevant to the use of descriptive and inferential statistics. The bulk of your effort will be spent digesting data from the studies included in the text.

LEARNING OUTCOMES

On completion of this chapter, you should be able to do the following:

- Differentiate between descriptive and inferential statistics.
- State the purposes of descriptive statistics.
- Identify the levels of measurement in a study.
- Describe a frequency distribution.
- List measures of central tendency and their use.
- List measures of variability and their use.
- State the purpose of inferential statistics.
- Explain the concept of probability as it applies to the analysis of sample data.
- Distinguish between a type I and type II error and its effect on a study's outcome.
- Distinguish between parametric and nonparametric tests.
- List some commonly used statistical tests and their purposes.
- Critically appraise the statistics used in published research studies.
- Evaluate the strength and quality of the evidence provided by the findings of a research study and determine applicability to practice.

If you are just learning about statistical analysis or are struggling to remember all of the new terms and where you would use a specific analysis, skip to the end of this chapter and complete the optional flash card activity.

Activity 1

Match the level of measurement found in Column B with the appropriate example(s) in Column A. (The levels of measurement in Column B will be used more than once. Table 16-1 from the text can assist you.)

Column A

1. _______ Amount of emesis
2. _______ Scores on the ACT, SAT, or GRE
3. _______ Height or weight
4. _______ Gender
5. _______ Satisfaction with nursing care
6. _______ Use or nonuse of contraception
7. _______ Class ranking
8. _______ Number of feet or meters walked
9. _______ Blood type
10. _______ Body temperature measured with centigrade thermometer
11. _______ Body temperature measured with Kelvin thermometer

Column B

a. Nominal
b. Ordinal
c. Interval
d. Ratio

Activity 2

If you have taken a course in statistics, you are familiar with the statistical notation used to refer to specific types of descriptive statistics. This activity will serve as a quick review. If you have not yet taken a statistics course, this exercise will provide you with enough information to recognize some of the statistical notations.

Column A

1. _______ Measure of central tendency used with interval or ratio data
2. _______ Abbreviation for the number of measures in a given data set (the measures may be individual people or some smaller piece of data like blood pressure readings)
3. _______ Measure of variation that shows the lowest and highest number in a set
4. _______ The percentage of cases a given score exceeds
5. _______ Old abbreviation for the mean
6. _______ Marks the "score" where 50% of the scores are higher and 50% are lower
7. _______ Describes a distribution characterized by a tail
8. _______ Abbreviation for standard deviation
9. _______ 68% of the values in a normal distribution fall between +1 of this statistic
10. _______ Very unstable measure
11. _______ The values that occur most frequently in a data set
12. _______ Describes a set of data with a standard deviation of 3 when compared with a set of data with a standard deviation of 12

Column B

a. X
b. N
c. Mode
d. Median
e. Range
f. Standard deviation
g. more homogeneous
h. skewed
i. percentile
j. SD

Activity 3

Read the following excerpts from specific studies included in your textbook. Identify both the independent and dependent variable(s) and indicate what level of measurement would apply. You may find the Critical Thinking Decision Path in the textbook to be helpful in answering these questions.

1. "All tests of significance were two-tailed with an alpha level of 0.01 to correct for the number of analyses performed and type I errors. Analyses were completed separately for parents and siblings. Pearson product-moment correlations and standard regressions with forward entry were conducted to examine parents' and siblings' reports of demographic and cancer-related variables in relation to their reported levels of psychological distress, life satisfaction, PTG, and coping strategies." (Turner-Sack et al., 2016)

   a. Name the variable of interest.

   b. Identify the level of measurement of this variable.

2. "Correlations were used to test the relationships of the SCS subscales with bereaved mothers' and fathers' grief (despair, detachment, disorganization), mental health (depression and PTSD) and personal growth at T1 and T2. Multiple regression analyses were used to test whether these relationships changed when the influence of race/ethnicity and religion were controlled. A priori power analysis showed that a sample size of 115 would provide sufficient power (≥80%) to detect an adjusted R2 of 0.02 representing a medium effect and with alpha set at. 05." (Hawthorne et al., 2016)

   a. Name the independent variable(s).

   b. Name the dependent variable(s).

   c. Identify the level of measurement of the independent variable.

3. "In 28 of the 35 participating families, the survivor and one of his or her parents participated, resulting in 28 matched survivor–parent dyads. Correlations for matched dyads are presented in Table 4. Parents' psychological distress was negatively correlated with their survivor child's active coping ($r = -0.53$, $p < 0.01$)." (Turner-Sack et al., 2016)

   a. What is a dyad? Why do the authors address this concept?

   b. What does this test measure?

Activity 4

Use the list of terms in column B to complete the items in Column A in this activity. (Some terms may be used more than once.)

Column A

1. _____ The ____________________________ states that there is no difference between the groups in the study or no association between the variables under study. Its usefulness to a study is that it is the only relationship that can be tested through the use of statistical tools.

2. _____ Analysis of variance (ANOVA) is an example of the use of ____________________________.

3. _____ It is impossible to prove that the ____________________________ is true.

4. _____ The tendency for statistics to fluctuate from one sample to another is known as the ____________________________.

5. _____, _____ The term ____________________________ refers to a characteristic of the population, whereas the term ____________________________ refers to a characteristic of a sample drawn from a population.

6. _____ When investigators are studying the association between variables, they often will use statistics that measure ______________________.

7. _____, _____ ____________________________ occurs when the investigator does not find statistical significance but a real difference exists in the world. A(n) ____________________________ occurs when the investigator concludes that there is a real (statistically significant) difference but, in reality, there is no difference.

8. _____ The relative frequency of an event in repeated trials under similar conditions is known as ____________________________ and provides the theoretical basis for inferential statistics.

9. _____ A statistically significant finding based on a change of 3 mm Hg in systolic blood pressure in a sample of healthy individuals likely would have little ____________________________.

10. _____ ____________________________ refer(s) to those tools used when data are collected at the ordinal or nominal level of measurement.

11. _____ When a finding is tested and found to be unlikely to have happened by chance, the investigators report ____________________________ for that particular finding.

12. _____ When a probability level is calculated as $p < .05$ and the investigator had set the alpha level of significance at 0.05, the investigator must reject the ____________________________ and accept the ______________________.

Column B

a. ANOVA
b. Correlation
c. Nonparametric statistics
d. Null hypothesis
e. Parameter
f. Parametric statistics
g. Practical significance
h. Probability
i. Research hypothesis
j. Sampling error
k. Statistic
l. Statistical significance
m. Type I error
n. Type II error

Activity 5

Using the studies in Appendices A through D in the textbook, answer the following questions regarding the use of descriptive and inferential statistics in each study. Once again, use Tables 16-3 and 16-4 and Figures 16-2 and 16-3 of the textbook.

1. Were descriptive statistics used in the study?
   a. Nyamathi et al.
   b. Hawthorne et al.
   c. van Dijk et al.
   d. Turner-Sack et al.

2. What data were summarized or explained through the use of the descriptive statistics described in your textbook?
   a. Nyamathi et al.
   b. Hawthorne et al.
   c. van Dijk et al.
   d. Turner-Sack et al.

3. Were the descriptive statistics used appropriately?
   a. Nyamathi et al.
   b. Hawthorne et al.
   c. van Dijk et al.
   d. Turner-Sack et al.

4. Did any of the four studies rely more heavily on the use of descriptive statistics than the others? If so, why do you think this occurred?

5. Now turn to the inferential statistics. Which of the four studies in the appendices used some type of inferential statistic to manage the data?
   a. Nyamathi et al.
   b. Hawthorne et al.
   c. van Dijk et al.
   d. Turner-Sack et al.

6. What inferential statistical tools described by your textbook were used in the studies?
   a. Nyamathi et al.
   b. Hawthorne et al.
   c. van Dijk et al.
   d. Turner-Sack et al.

Optional Flash Card Activity 6

If you are new to statistics or need a refresher course, before you start any of the activities for Chapter 16, make life easier for yourself—create tools that will provide a shortcut. Create a set of reference cards that can also serve as flashcards.

Create your own set of "statistical assistants." Once the cards are finished, carry them with you to the library, or set them on the desk while working on the Internet. Use them when reading research reports. Before long, you will be able to read a piece of research without referring to the stack of statistical assistants, and you will master the best shortcut of all: memorizing the statistical notation. Flipping through the pages of a book looking for a statistical symbol before you can evaluate the use of the statistic will no longer be required.

Gather the following supplies: package of 3 × 5 index cards, preferably lined on one side; pens or a combination of pens and highlighters with different colors; one broad-tipped, black-ink marker; your textbook turned to Chapter 16, Tables 16-1, 16-3, and 16-4.

1. Make three key cards first. On one of the 3 × 5 cards, on the side without lines, use the broad-tipped black marker and write "INFERENTIAL STATISTICAL TECHNIQUES—relationship" and on another write "INFERENTIAL STATISTICAL TECHNIQUES—difference." Take the third 3 × 5 card and write "DESCRIPTIVE TECHNIQUES" on the unlined side.

2. Turn the *inferential statistics—relationship* card over to the lined side. With one of the colored pens, write on the left side of the card the following list:

   2 variables; interval measure
   2 variables; nominal or ordinal
   >2 variables; interval measure
   >2 variables; nominal or ordinal

   Next to the descriptors at the left, write the tests used for each type of data.

3. Turn the *inferential statistics—difference* card over to the lined side. With one of the colored pens, write on the left side of the card the following list:

   2 groups; interval measure
   2 groups; nominal or ordinal
   1 group; interval measure
   1 group; nominal or ordinal

   Next to the descriptors at the left, write the tests used for each type of data.

4. Do the same with the *descriptive statistics* card. Write on the left side of the card the following list:

   nominal measurement
   ordinal measurement
   interval measurement
   ratio measurement

   Next to the descriptors at the left, write the tests used for each type of data.

5. Each line of the key card should be in a different color. Next, create a stack of statistical assistants.

6. Take a blank card. On the front of each card (unlined side) write the full name of one of the statistical tools using the broad-tipped black marker (or whatever marker was used to write on the front of the key card) (example: *mean*).

7. Turn the card over and write the information that corresponds to the appropriate category on the key card on the appropriate line using the appropriate color. If you need assistance with choosing the appropriate information to put on each line, refer to Tables 16-1, 16-3, and 16-4; the descriptions of each test in your textbook; and the Critical Thinking Decision Path in Chapter 16 of the text. For example, the lined side of *mean* would read as follows:

   Mathematical average of all scores
   Interval or ratio data
   Most-used measure of central tendency, often used in tests of significance
   Affected by every score, extreme scores can lead to big changes
   Symbol: (see text)
   Best point for summarizing interval or ratio data

8. These cards will fit into an envelope or any of the small plastic cases that can be purchased from the local bookstore. They will slip into a bookbag, briefcase, or backpack with ease.

POSTTEST

1. Two outpatient clinics measured patient waiting time as one indicator of effectiveness. The mean and standard deviation of waiting time in minutes is reported here. Which outpatient clinic would you prefer, assuming that all other things are equal? Explain your answer.

	Clinic 1	Clinic 2
Mean (in minutes)	40	25
Standard deviation (in minutes)	10	45

2. You are responsible for ordering a new supply of hospital gowns for your unit. Which measure of central tendency would be the most useful in your decision-making? Explain your answer.

3. Matching exercise for measures of central tendency: Draw a line connecting the measure of central tendency with the correct description.

Mode	Most frequent score
Median	Arithmetical average, most stable
Mean	Middle score

Use the terms in Column B to fill in the blanks in Column A for the following statements in questions 4 to 9. Not all terms will be used and some terms may be used more than once.

	Column A	Column B
4. _____, _____, _____	A ____________________ distribution is said to have __________ or ____________ skew.	a. χ^2
		b. Hypothesis
		c. Inferential
5. _____	We use inferential statistics to test a(n) ______________.	d. Negative
6. _____, _____, _____	______________ ________________ like the normal curve are the basis for all ______________ statistics.	e. Nonsymmetrical
		f. Null hypothesis
		g. Positive
		h. Sampling distributions
7. _____, _____	The __________ ____________ states that there is no relationship between the variables.	i. Type II error
		j. Type I error
8. _____, _____	If a researcher accepts a null hypothesis that is *not* true, this is a(n) ________ ________ error.	
9. _____	A statistical test for differences in proportions is the _______ test.	

10. Identify the components of the following statistical test result: χ^2 (6, n = 213) = 33.0, $p < .0001$. Match the component with its correct name.

_____ χ^2	a. Sample size
_____ 6	b. Degrees of freedom
_____ $n = 213$	c. Chi-square symbol
_____ 33.0	d. Probability level
_____ $p < .0001$	e. Chi-square test statistic

REFERENCES

Hawthorne, D. M., Youngblut, J. M., & Brooten, D. (2016). Parent spirituality, grief, and mental health at 1 and 3 months after their infant's/child's death in an intensive care unit. *Journal of Pediatric Nursing, 31*(1), 73-80.

Nyamathi, A., Salem, B. E., Zhang, S., Farabee, D., Hall, B., Khalilifard, F., & Leake, B. (2016). Nursing care management, peer coaching, and hepatitis A and B vaccine completion among homeless men recently released on parole. *Nursing Research, 64*, 177-189.

Turner-Sack, A. M., Menna, R., Setchell, S. R., Maan, C., & Cataudella, D. (2016). Psychological functioning, post traumatic growth, and coping in parents and siblings of adolescent cancer survivors. *Oncology Nursing Forum, 43*, 48-57.

van Dijk, J. F. M., Vervoort, S. C. J. M., van Wijck, A. J. M., Kalkman, C. J., & Schuurmans, M. J. (2016). Postoperative patients' perspective on rating pain: A qualitative study. *International Journal of Nursing Studies, 53*, 260-269.

17 Understanding Research Findings

INTRODUCTION

As the last sections of a research report, the Results and Discussions sections answer the question "So what?" In other words, it is in these two sections that the investigator "makes sense" of the research, critically synthesizes the data, ties them to a theoretical framework, and builds on a body of knowledge. These two sections are a very important part of the research report because they describe the generalizability of the findings and offer recommendations for further research. Well-written, clear, and concise Results and Discussions sections provide valuable information for nursing practice. Conversely, poorly written Results and Discussions sections will leave a reader bewildered, confused, and wondering how or if the findings are relevant to nursing.

LEARNING OUTCOMES

On completion of this chapter, you should be able to do the following:

- Discuss the difference between the Results and Discussion sections of a research study.
- Determine if findings are objectively discussed.
- Identify the format and components of the Results section.
- Describe how tables and figures are used in a research report.
- List the criteria of a meaningful table.
- Identify the purpose and components of the Discussion section.
- Discuss the importance of including generalizability and limitations of a study in the report.
- Determine the purpose of including recommendations in the study report.
- Discuss how the strength, quality, and consistency of evidence provided by the findings are related to a study's results, limitations, generalizability, and applicability to practice.

Activity 1

Knowing what information to look for and where to find it in the Results and Discussions sections of a research report will enable you to interpret the research findings and critique research reports. Identify the section in which the following information from the research report may be found. Put an *R* in the blank space if the information would be found in the Results section and a *D* if the information would be found in the Discussion section.

1. ________ Tables/figures to present large amounts of data
2. ________ Limitations of the study
3. ________ Analysis of each question or hypothesis
4. ________ Strength and quality of the evidence
5. ________ Statistical tests used to analyze the data
6. ________ Statistical software program
7. ________ Recommendations for practice and future research

Activity 2

Match the term in Column B with the appropriate definition in Column A.

Column A

1. _____ Values that quantify the probable value range within which a population parameter is expected to lie
2. _____ Inferences that the data are representative of similar phenomena in a population beyond the study's sample
3. _____ The results, conclusions, interpretations, recommendations, and implications for future research and nursing practice of a study
4. _____ The researchers' suggestions for the study's application to practice, theory, and further research
5. _____ Threats to a study's internal or external validity

Column B

a. Findings
b. Generalizability
c. Limitations
d. Confidence interval
e. Recommendations

Activity 3

For questions 1 through 6, answer *true* (T) or *false* (F).

1. _______ Rarely should one study be a recommendation for action.
2. _______ If the results of a study are not supported statistically or are only partially supported, the study is irrelevant and should not have been published.
3. _______ Good tables repeat what the researchers have written in the text.
4. _______ The researchers should respond objectively to the results in the discussion of the findings.
5. _______ All studies have limitations.
6. _______ Statistically significant findings are the sole means for establishing a study's merit.

POSTTEST

The Results and Discussion sections are the researcher's opportunity to examine the logic of the hypotheses or research questions posed, the theoretical framework, the methods, and the analysis of the study. Using the following criteria, review and critique the Results, Discussion, and Conclusions sections of the study by Hawthorne et al. (2016) found in Appendix D in the text.

1. In the Results section, the authors list some of the demographic data in the text and then refer to Table 1. Table 1 contains much information that was not included in the text. Please choose the best explanation for the difference.

   a. The data contained in the table but not mentioned in the text did not reach statistical significance and did not need to be mentioned.

   b. A good table does not simply repeat information given in the text; rather, it economizes and supplements the text.

   c. The information not included in the first paragraph of the Results section but contained in the table was included in full in the remaining Results and Discussion sections.

   d. Journal style and space limitations prohibit the inclusion of descriptive statistics in the text.

2. How did the authors present the results of their study?

   a. The results begin with a written summary of the demographic data and a corresponding data table, then they report on the findings of the independent and dependent variables in sections mirroring the presentation of these variables in the Methods section. Finally they interpret the results in the Discussion section.

   b. The authors presented the most statistically important findings first, followed by other significant results.

   c. The authors presented each research hypothesis, then the statistical software package and type of statistical analysis, and finally they reported the results of all tests where the null hypothesis was rejected. They included figures and tables with all corresponding data, confidence intervals, and level of statistical significance.

   d. This was a qualitative study, and the data included quotes and text but only small amounts of data—namely, the demographic information.

3. Which of the following tests were used to analyze the data presented? Choose all that apply.

   a. General linear mixed model

   b. Chi-square analysis

   c. Correlation

   d. Multiple regression analyses

4. If tables or figures are used, (A) do they supplement and economize the text, (B) do they have precise titles and headings, and (C) are they not repetitious of the text? a. Yes b. No

5. If the data are supported, does the investigator provide a discussion of how the theoretical framework was supported? a. Yes b. No

6. Does the investigator attempt to identify the study's weaknesses—that is, threats to internal and external validity—and strengths, as well as suggest possible solutions for the research area? a. Yes b. No

7. Does the researcher discuss the study's clinical relevance? a. Yes b. No

8. Are any recommendations for future research stated or implied? a. Yes b. No

REFERENCE

Hawthorne, D. M., Youngblut, J. M., & Brooten, D. (2016). Parent spirituality, grief, and mental health at 1 and 3 months after their infant's/child's death in an intensive care unit. *Journal of Pediatric Nursing, 31*(1), 73-80.

18 Appraising Quantitative Research

INTRODUCTION

Chapter 18 in the textbook includes two thorough critiques of two quantitative studies. The first study critiqued is one by Bakas et al. (2015) that examined the effectiveness of an intervention (Telephone Assessment and Skill-Building Kit [TASK II]) for enabling stroke family caregivers to build skills based on assessment of their own needs. The second critique is of a study by Zeleníková et al. (2016) that examined predictors of caregivers' perceptions of the suffering of patients with a primary malignant brain tumor and the extent that perceived suffering predicts caregivers' burden and depression. The results in Chapter 18 are complete critiques of two separate studies.

Both of these critiques reflect the level of analysis desired for an article that the registered nurse had decided was relevant to practice. If you want to produce a critique at this level of thoroughness, it will take time. It would not be uncommon for a novice reader of research to use 2 to 3 hours (maybe more) to complete such a critique. Usually novice readers of research find the task tedious and, not infrequently, difficult. The more often you read and critique studies in this manner, the easier (and more interesting) reading research becomes. The easier it becomes, the more quickly you can complete a critique. To get started, you just have to pick an article, dive in, and do it.

One way of getting started is to commit to work to improve your critiquing skills. For example, you could commit to finding one research study every week that is relevant to an area of nursing you are interested in or a question you have related to nursing practice, and then critique that article using the steps outlined in the textbook. At the end of a year, you could have read almost four dozen studies.

As mentioned earlier, this level of reading and critiquing is most often used when you have a reasonable expectation that a specific study will be useful in your professional practice. But not all relevant articles will be found in the journals that are devoted specifically to your area of clinical expertise. Often you may find yourself searching through several electronic databases or numerous journals to find studies that can be useful. When you do find a study that appears to be practice relevant, you need to assess the article quickly so you can decide whether you should be spending the time to critically appraise the study.

LEARNING OUTCOMES

On completion of this chapter, you should be able to do the following:

- Identify the purpose of the critical appraisal process.
- Describe the criteria for each step of the critical appraisal process.
- Describe the strengths and weaknesses of a research report.
- Assess the strength, quality, and consistency of evidence provided by a quantitative research report.
- Discuss applicability of the findings of a research report for evidence-based nursing practice.
- Conduct a critique of a research report.

Activity 1

This quick reading of articles demands the reader consider the same aspects of a study that you would consider if completing a more detailed critique, but in a more superficial manner. This type of reading is called "inspectional reading" (Adler & Van Doren, 1972). Mastering inspectional reading is essential but is often overlooked in regard to analytical skills. Often, professional reading must be squeezed into a small window of available time. Improving your quick reading skills will help you sort through the reading required to maintain and expand your knowledge base.

But what is this inspectional reading? It is the second level in a set of skills described by Adler and Van Doren (1972). The first skill is elementary reading, which is usually accomplished very early in formal education. Level two is inspectional reading. Level three is analytical reading, where the reader is trying very hard to understand what the author is attempting to share, and is the level of reading required to produce a critique of a research study. Level four is syntopical reading, which requires intense effort to synthesize ideas from many sources.

Inspectional reading has two components. The first is called "systematic skimming" and the second is called "superficial reading."

Systematic skimming is the first thing anyone should do when approaching a research study. It requires only a few minutes to skim an article—but it may take up to an hour if you are skimming a complete book. Let's assume that you are going to skim a hard copy of a research study.

- Read the title and the abstract.
- Read the biographical information about the authors/researchers.
- Read the Conclusions section.
- Ask yourself the following question: "Is the clinical question addressed in the study similar to the clinical question that I have?" Or more specifically, are the components of your PICO or PECO or PS question similar to that of the study? Remember PICO includes the patients/population, intervention, comparison, and outcome(s); PECO includes the patients/population, exposure, comparison, and outcome(s); and PS includes the patients/population and the situation. If your answer is "no," it is likely OK to put this study down and move on to the next study or search for another study. If your answer "unsure" or "yes," proceed to superficial reading of the article.

Superficial reading requires that you read the article from beginning to end without stopping. Try your best not to take notes, highlight (hide your highlighter so you won't even be tempted), or use a dictionary to understand words that you do not know. Try not to even stop to think "I wonder what they meant by that?" The key to this step is ... just read.

When you have completed the article, take a deep breath and ask yourself these questions:

- What do I remember about the study? The question? The methods? The results? The discussion?
- Was the research design experimental, nonexperimental, or qualitative?
- Where would the study fit in terms of level of evidence?
- Did anything in the study raise any ethical questions?
- Does it fit with my clinical question? If the answer is "no," again it's probably time to move on to the next article. If the answer is "maybe" put it in a "come-back-to-later" stack. If the answer is "yes," proceed to more detailed reading while writing down notes that would be necessary to complete a critical appraisal, such as the two examples found in Chapter 18.

Activity 2

The article by Nyamathi et al. (2015) in Appendix A of the textbook has been used for several activities throughout this study guide. However, it is quite possible that you have not read it completely, at one time, from beginning to end. For this activity, consider the following scenario:

You currently work as a registered nurse in a public health department. As part of involvement in your unit's journal club, every other month you are responsible for identifying a research study that is relevant to practice. To help you find a relevant research study, you have been asking your colleagues what they think is the most important issue on the unit for patients. The issue of hepatitis vaccination among homeless men is identified as one of the priority issue areas.

Now, read the study by Nyamathi et al., practicing the use of systematic skimming and inspectional reading strategies. When you have done so, answer the questions that follow.

Systematic skimming:

- What do you know about the authors/researchers?
- How does the clinical question addressed in the study compare with the clinical question in the scenario?

Superficial reading:

- What do I remember about the study? The question? The methods? The results? The discussion?
- Was the research design experimental, nonexperimental, or qualitative?
- Where would the study fit in terms of level of evidence?
- Did anything in the study raise any ethical questions?
- Does it fit with my clinical question?

Activity 3

Often in practice, nurses are asked to summarize their critical appraisal of a research study within a very short time frame (i.e., 2-3 minutes). Consider the same scenario as in Activity 2 and the study by Nyamathi et al. (2015) in Appendix A. Keeping in mind that this study has been used for several activities throughout the textbook and study guide, review the study in terms of the critical appraisal criteria Table 18-1 provided in Chapter 18 of the textbook.

In no more than five sentences, summarize the following for the study by Nyamathi et al. (2015). (Note: Refer to the "Conclusions/Implications/Recommendations" and "Application to Nursing Practice" sections from the two critical appraisal examples in Chapter 18 as a guide.)

- Population (or sample)
- Type of study (i.e., level of evidence)
- Strengths and limitations
- Results (i.e., "Is there a difference between the study groups?" "Is the difference statistically significant?")
- Applicability to practice

POSTTEST

There is no posttest for this chapter. Enjoy the break!

REFERENCES

Adler, M. J., & Van Doren, C. (1972). *How to read a book.* New York, NY: Simon & Schuster.

Nyamathi, A., Salem, B. E., Zhang, S., Farabee, D., Hall, B., Khalilifard, F., & Leake, B. (2015). Nursing care management, peer coaching, and hepatitis A and B vaccine completion among homeless men recently released on parole. *Nursing Research, 64*(3), 177-189.

19 Strategies and Tools for Developing an Evidence-Based Practice

INTRODUCTION

Maintaining a clinical practice that incorporates new evidence can be challenging. This chapter will assist you in becoming a more efficient and effective reader of the literature by providing you with a few important tools to assist you in determining the merits of a study for your practice and patients.

LEARNING OUTCOMES

After reading this chapter, you should be able to do the following:

- Identify the key elements of a focused clinical question.
- Discuss the use of databases to search the literature.
- Screen a research article for relevance and validity.
- Critically appraise study results and apply the findings to practice.
- Make clinical decisions based on evidence from the literature combined with clinical expertise and patient preferences.

Activity 1

Using the PICO format to organize a clinical question is helpful to the nurse who is searching for the best-available evidence. In addition to determining major search terms, the PICO format also helps the nurse determine the clinical category to which a research study belongs. Follow the instructions below.

A. Put the following clinical questions into PICO format. (Note: Depending on the questions being asked, in some studies there may be no "C" or comparison).

B. Identify which clinical category you would expect the study to belong to.

Therapy (T)
Diagnosis (D)
Prognosis (P)
Causation/Harm (C/H)

1. In older adults, do measures of the frequency and duration of social interactions predict mortality?

a. P ____________________

____

b. I ____________________

____

c. C ____________________

____

d. O ____________________

____

e. Clinical Category: ____________________

2. Is hyperbaric oxygen treatment more effective than wound coverage by cultured cells for diabetic foot ulcers in patients without arterial insufficiency?

   a. P ______________________________

   ____

   b. I ______________________________

   ____

   c. C ______________________________

   ____

   d. O ______________________________

   ____

   e. Clinical Category: ______________________________

3. What is the accuracy of self report measures in screening for substance abuse among adolescents in a hospital-based clinic?

   a. P ______________________________

   ____

   b. I ______________________________

   ____

   c. C ______________________________

   ____

   d. O ______________________________

   ____

   e. Clinical Category: ______________________________

4. Is there an association between the risk of childhood brain or central nervous system cancers and residential exposure to low level radio frequency radiation from smart meters?

   a. P ______________________________

   ____

   b. I ______________________________

   ____

   c. C ______________________________

   ____

   d. O ______________________________

   ____

   e. Clinical Category: ______________________________

Activity 2: Web-Based Activity

As mentioned earlier, determining the clinical category of a research study will help in your search for the best-available evidence. Access the following online bibliographic databases and list the clinical category filters for each database.

1. CINAHL

2. PubMed (Medline)—Use search bar to complete initial search. Once search results have appeared, look to the left-hand tool bar; under "Article Types," select "Customize" to see menu to filter your results.

4. PubMed (Medline)—click on "Clinical Queries" on left side of the home page.

4. Based on the clinical category filters for each of the previous bibliographic databases, which database do you think would provide you the most efficient search if you were able to identify the clinical category of the PICO question you were searching for?

Activity 3

Match the term in Column B with the appropriate interpretation in Column A.

Column A

1. _______ Number of adults who need to receive the RTS,S vaccine in order to prevent one adult from being diagnosed with a new malaria infection
2. _______ Risk of a new malaria infection being 0.96 times less for adults who receive the RTS,S vaccine than for those who do not receive the RTS,S vaccine
3. _______ Rapid screening tests being 96% accurate in detecting the proportion of patients with a negative test as not having malaria
4. _______ Number of patients diagnosed with malaria
5. _______ Malaria being 4.8 times more likely to be reported among Swedish children ages 1 to 6 years than other age groups
6. _______ 78% of patients presenting to an outpatient clinic with a positive rapid screening test having malaria
7. _______ Percentage of patients diagnosed with malaria
8. _______ 1% of adults who receive the RTS,S vaccine do not develop a new malaria infection
9. _______ Rapid screening tests being 95% accurate in detecting the proportion of patients with positive tests as having malaria
10. _______ 95% of patients presenting to an outpatient clinic with a negative rapid screening test will not have malaria
11. _______ RTS,S vaccination reduces new malaria infections by 4% relative to not receiving the vaccination

Column B

a. Continuous variable
b. Categorical variable
c. Relative risk
d. Relative risk reduction
e. Odds ratio
f. Absolute risk reduction
g. Number needed to treat
h. Sensitivity
i. Specificity
j. Positive predictive value
k. Negative predictive value

Activity 4

As an RN working in an outpatient primary care office, you are concerned with the effectiveness of tobacco cessation interventions. Because you find a difference in smoking rates between two primary care offices in different neighborhoods, you perform a literature review to see what factors can affect rates of tobacoo use . You retrieve the randomized controlled trial by Hass et al. (2015). The following is a summary of the design and findings. Use this information to answer questions 1 to 6.

Setting: 13 primary care practices in the Boston area.

Sample: n = 707 low SES (socioeconomic status) adult smokers

Methods: Smokers were identified through the electronic health record (EHR) and contacted via interactive voice response platform, following contact and informed consent, patients were randomized to control or intervention groups in batches based on the date of their clinic visit.

Intervention: Intervention program that included (1) telephone-based motivational counseling, .(2) free nicotine replacement therapy (NRT), (3) access to community-based referrals to address sociocontextual mediators of tobacco use, and (4) integration of all these components into their normal health care through the EHR system. Self report measures of past-7-day tobacco abstinence 9 months after randomization ("quitting"), assessed by automated caller or blinded study staff.

Control: Usual care.

Findings: The intervention group had a higher quit rate than the usual care group (17.8% vs 8.1%; odds ratio, 2.5; 95% CI 1.5-4.0; number needed to treat, 10). We examined whether use of intervention components was associated with quitting among individuals in the intervention group: individuals who participated in the telephone counseling were more likely to quit than those who did not (21.2% vs 10.4%; P<.001). There was no difference in quitting by use of NRT. Quitting did not differ by a request for a community referral, but individuals who used their referral were more likely to quit than those who did not (43.6% vs 15.3%; P<.001).

1. How was the outcome variable measured? Was it measured as a (a) continuous or (b) discrete variable?

2. What is the null value of the outcome measure used to interpret the confidence interval (CI)?

3. How would you interpret the CI?

4. The results of the study are expressed as an odds ratio (OR). Interpret the OR and determine if it is statistically significant.

5. Interpret the number needed treat (NNT). How was it calculated? Is the NNT clinically useful?

6. How would you apply the results of this study to the clinical situation?

Activity 5

You are a nurse working in an outpatient pediatric practice. After working for several years, you start to wonder why it seems that more of your pediatric patients are developing obesity despite seeing only soda with artificial sweeteners consumed by parents. Out of curiosity, you perform a quick literature review to see if the evidence supports your observations. You retrieve the longitudinal study by Azad et al. (2016). The following is a summary of the design and findings Use this information to answer questions 1 to 6.

Setting: Canada

Sample: n = 3,033 mother-infant dyads

Outcomes: Maternal consumption of artificially sweetened beverages during pregnancy (food frequency questionnaire), infant body mass index (z score) at 1 year of age.

Findings: The mean (SD) age of the 3033 pregnant women was 32.4 (4.7) years, and their mean (SD) BMI was 24.8 (5.4). The mean (SD) infant BMI *z* score at 1 year of age was 0.19 (1.05), and 5.1% of infants were overweight. More than a quarter of women (29.5%) consumed artificially sweetened beverages during pregnancy, including 5.1% who reported daily consumption. Compared with no consumption, daily consumption of artificially sweetened beverages was associated with a 0.20-unit increase in infant BMI *z* score (adjusted 95% CI, 0.02-0.38) and a 2-fold higher risk of infant overweight at 1 year of age (adjusted odds ratio, 2.19; 95% CI, 1.23-3.88). These effects were not explained by maternal BMI, diet quality, total energy intake, or other obesity risk factors. There were no comparable associations for sugar-sweetened beverages.

1. What was the PICO question addressed in the clinical situation?

   P ____

   I ____

   C ____

   O ____

2. The question addressed in the study by Azad et al. (2016) was, "To determine whether maternal consumption of artificially sweetened beverages during pregnancy is associated with infant body mass index (BMI [calculated as weight in kilograms divided by height in meters squared])".How does the PICO question in the clinical situation compare with the PICO question asked by Peterson et al. (2008)?

3. Based on the PICO question of the clinical situation and the question addressed in the study by Azad et al. (2016), what clinical category is being addressed? Structured tools are available to help you systematically appraise the strength and quality of evidence for a given category of a clinical question. Although many tools exist, the tools developed by the Centre for Evidence Based Medicine (http://www.cebm.net/critical-appraisal/) can help guide your critical appraisal of a prognostic study to critique the study by Azad et al. (2008).

4. Indicate whether each of the outcomes are *continuous variables* (C) or *discrete/dichotomous variables* (D).

   a. ________ daily consumption of artificially sweetened beverages

   b. ________ age of the pregnant women

   c. ________ infant BMI z score at 1 year

5. Interpret the study findings. Which findings are statistically significant? How can you tell?

6. How would you apply the results of this study to the clinical situation? Do the results warrant an evidence-based practice change?

POSTTEST

Determine whether each of the following statements is *true* (T) or *false* (F). If an item is false, revise it to make it a true statement.

1. ________ An experimental or quasiexperimental study design is usually used for the causation/harm category of clinical concern used by clinicians.
2. ________ Articles should be screened to determine if the setting and sample in the study are similar to my clinical situation.
3. ________ A confidence interval can provide the reader information about the statistical significance of the findings.
4. ________ *Specificity* is the term used to describe the proportion of individuals with a disease who test positive for it.
5. ________ A confidence interval does not provide the reader information about the clinical significance of the findings.
6. ________ The null value for continuous variables is 0.
7. ________ NNT is a useful measure for applying research findings to practice.
8. ________ *Prevalence* is a term used to describe the number that expresses the sensitivity, specificity, positive predictive value (PPV), and negative predictive value (NPV).

REFERENCES

Azad, M. B., Sharma, A. K., de Souza, R. J., et al. (2016). Association between artificially sweetened beverage consumption during pregnancy and infant body mass index. *JAMA Pediatrics, 170*(7), 662–670. doi:10.1001/jamapediatrics.2016.0301.

Haas, J. S., Linder, J. A., Park, E. R., et al. (2015). Proactive tobacco cessation outreach to smokers of low socioeconomic status: a randomized clinical trial. *JAMA Internal Medicine, 175*(2), 218–226. doi:10.1001/jamainternmed.2014.6674.

20 Developing an Evidence-Based Practice

INTRODUCTION

Engaging in evidence-based practice has become an expected standard in the delivery of health care services. Although there are concentrated efforts on methods to facilitate the translation of research findings into practice, nurses can engage in evidence-based practice through the development, implementation, and evaluation of evidence-based changes in practice. You have the ability to make positive changes in nursing practice using these tools. This chapter presents an overview of evidence-based practice and the process for applying evidence in practice to improve patient outcomes.

LEARNING OUTCOMES

On completion of this chapter, you should be able to do the following:

- Differentiate among conduct of nursing research, evidence-based practice, and translation science.
- Describe the steps of evidence-based practice.
- Describe strategies for implementing evidence-based practice changes.
- Identify steps for evaluating an evidence-based change in practice.
- Use research findings and other forms of evidence to improve the quality of care.

Activity 1

Although *translation science* and *evidence-based practice* are often associated, they are not exactly the same. Answer the following to help you differentiate between the two terms.

1. Identify the key differences between *translation science* and *evidence-based practice*. Mark each of the following as (a) translation science or (b) evidence-based practice.

    1. ________ Studying variables that affect knowledge uptake and use
    2. ________ The application of evidence in practice
    3. ________ Conscientious and judicious use of current best evidence in conjunction with clinical expertise and patient preference to guide health care decisions
    4. ________ May include promoting knowledge uptake and changing practitioner behavior
    5. ________ Strategies that address the systems of care, individual practitioners, senior leadership, and changing health care cultures

2. Identify the three major components of evidence-based practice.

    a. ____________________

    b. ____________________

    c. ____________________

Activity 2

Following are short descriptions of RN activities related to research. Each can be categorized as one of the following:

a. Conduct of research
b. Dissemination of research findings
c. Research utilization
d. Evidence-based practice

Place the letter (a, b, c, d) that best describes each activity in the space provided. (Some letters will be used more than once.)

1. _______ The RN submits an article to his or her health care agency's in-house practice newsletter about the research study he or she participated in.

2. _______ As a member of the health care team, the RN was involved with developing a plan of care for a patient using the findings from one meta-analysis and several research studies.

3. _______ Two RNs are involved with data collection for a study comparing two types of dressings for postoperative incisions.

4. _______ The RN has read about an intervention that will reduce the pain associated with the injection of a particular medication. After reviewing all of the variables, he or she decides that trying the intervention would be a good idea and proceeds to develop an implementation plan.

5. _______ Marie has been working with a faculty member on an independent study project. The two of them have decided to publish the results of their work.

6. _______ A journal club group composed of RNs, MDs, and NPs have identified a specific clinical question and plan to develop a practice guideline by the end of the year.

Activity 3

Number the following major steps of evidence-based practice in the correct sequence. Use the number 1 for the first step.

a. _______ Choose an approach to assess the quality of the individual research and strength of the body of evidence.

b. _______ Select a topic.

c. _______ Critique the research.

d. _______ Implement the evidence-based change in practice.

e. _______ Form a team.

f. _______ Evaluate the evidence-based change in practice.

g. _______ Identify evidence-based practice recommendations.

h. _______ Write the evidence-based practice standard.

i. _______ Retrieve the best-available evidence.

j. _______ Synthesize the evidence.

k. _______ Decide if a change in practice is warranted.

Activity 4

Fill in the blanks in Column A with the appropriate word(s) from Column B.

Column A

1. ________, ________ Clinical questions arise from different types of "triggers." ________________ triggers are identified by staff through quality improvement, risk surveillance, benchmarking data, financial data, or recurrent clinical problems, whereas ________________ triggers are ideas generated when staff read research, listen to scientific papers at research conferences, or encounter evidence-based practice guidelines published by federal agencies or specialty organizations.

2. ________ A team is responsible for the development, implementation, and evaluation of an evidence-based practice project. This team is likely to include ________________, who are key individuals who will be affected by the implementation of the evidence-based practice project and who are critical to its successful implementation.

3. ________, ________, ________ Formulating clinical questions assists in the retrieval of relevant research and related literature. PICO is one such effective approach to formulating clinical questions. Identify the four components of this acronym: P ________________; I ________________; C ________________; O ________________

Column B

a. Patient, population, or problem
b. Problem-focused
c. Stakeholders
d. Intervention/treatment
e. Knowledge-focused
f. Outcomes
g. Comparison intervention/treatment

Activity 5

Once evidence-based practice recommendations have been developed from the critique and synthesis of the best available evidence, it is then important to determine if these recommendations should result in an evidence-based change in practice. Indicate *yes* (Y) or *no* (N) as to whether the following should be considered in making this decision. The extent to which:

1. ________ there is consistency in findings across studies/guidelines.
2. ________ the evidence was published in peer-reviewed journals.
3. ________ a significant number of studies/guidelines with sample characteristics similar to those to which the recommendations will be used.
4. ________ the studies support current practice.
5. ________ the authors of the studies and/or guidelines are well known in their field.
6. ________ feasibility exists for use in practice.

Activity 6

Although a practice change may be evidence based, its adoption depends on several factors. The answers to the following questions will help identify factors influencing the adoption of an evidence-based practice change.

1. According to Rogers' Diffusion of Innovation model, identify two factors that influence the adoption of evidence-based practice innovations.

   a. ____

   b. ____

2. Match the term in Column B with the appropriate interpretation in Column A.

Column A		Column B
a. ______	Practitioners within the local group setting who are expert clinicians, are passionate about the innovation, are committed to improving quality of care, and have a positive working relationship with other health professionals	1. Audit and feedback
b. ______	Key individual or group of individuals who will be directly or indirectly affected by the implementation of the evidence-based change in practice	2. Opinion leader
c. ______	Ongoing auditing of performance indicators, aggregating data into reports, and discussing the findings with practitioners during an evidence-based change in practice	3. Change champion
d. ______	Practitioner who is considered by the local group as being dedicated, competent, and trusted to evaluate new information in the context of group norms	4. Stakeholders

3. Determine whether each of the following strategies have seemed to have a positive effect on promoting the use of evidence-based practices. Place a "Y" next to those you think have a positive effect and an "N" next to those you do not think have a positive effect on evidence-based practices.

   a. Mass media ____

   b. Change champions ____

   c. Didactic education ____

   d. Opinion leaders ____

POSTTEST

Retrieve the article by Dockham et al. (2016) shown in the reference list. Based on the article, answer the following questions about evidence-based practice change.

1. What was the overall topic of the evidence-based practice change?

2. Describe some of the members of the evidence-based practice team and the types of collaborations they built to support this study.

3. Who, if anyone, would you identify as "stakeholders" in the evidence-based practice team?

4. Was the best available evidence retrieved? If so, which strategies were used?

5. What was the approach for grading the quality of the individual evidence and strength of the body of evidence?

6. Was the research evidence (existing clinical practice guidelines, systematic reviews [including meta-analyses and/or meta-syntheses], and primary sources/individual research studies) critiqued?

7. Was the research evidence synthesized? What were the evidence-based practice change recommendations?

8. Was the evidence-based practice change written in detail?

9. How was the decision to make the evidence-based practice change supported?

10. Is a method for evaluating the feasibility of the evidence-based practice change identified?

11. Was the evidence-based practice change evaluated? Was it successful?

12. What were the strategies used by the evidence-based change team to promote the adoption of the evidence-based practice change?

REFERENCE

Dockham, B., Schafenacker, A., Yoon, H., Ronis, D. L., Kershaw, T., Titler, M. G., & Northouse, L. (2016). Implementation of a psychoeducational program for cancer survivors and family caregivers at a cancer support community affiliate: A pilot effectiveness study. *Cancer Nursing, 39*(3), 169-180.

21 Quality Improvement

INTRODUCTION

We've all had moments as nurses or as patients where we can see how the efficiency of a health care process could improve or how safety could be increased. As nurses, we are on the front lines providing care and we have the tools to effect changes in health care that can make a meaningful difference for our patients. Not every improvement in care is due to a large scientific study, and in fact many improvements in the quality of care come from small changes based on quality improvement (QI). QI uses data to improve the quality and safety of health care by monitoring outcomes of care processes. QI employs improvement methods to continuously aim for better care by designing and testing changes. QI complements evidence-based practice (EBP) and research efforts to improve care.

Efficiency, access, safety, timeliness, and patient-centeredness problems in clinical settings are ideal candidates for quality improvement solutions. Nurses play key roles in QI activities, and as a nurse you will probably be involved in QI activities in your professional capacity. With a basic understanding of QI, you will be prepared to play your role in improving care for your patients.

LEARNING OUTCOMES

On completion of this chapter, you should be able to do the following:

- Discuss the characteristics of quality health care defined by the Institute of Medicine.
- Compare the characteristics of the major quality improvement (QI) models used in health care.
- Identify two databases used to report health care organizations' performance to promote consumer choice and guide clinical QI activities.
- Describe the relationship between nursing-sensitive quality indicators and patient outcomes.
- Describe the steps in the improvement process and determine appropriate QI tools to use in each phase of the improvement process.
- List four themes for improvement to apply to the unit where you work.
- Describe ways that nurses can lead QI projects in clinical settings.
- Use the SQUIRE guidelines to critique a journal article reporting the results of a QI project.

Activity 1

Quality improvement efforts are one part of the wider effort to improve patient care. QI, evidence-based practice, and research have many similarities that may be confusing. In this exercise, we'll build a table of the major differences in QI, EBP, and research based on what you have learned in Chapter 21 and throughout this textbook. Please fill in each column after reviewing the final chapter in your book.

	Quality Improvement	Evidence-Based Practice	Research
Purpose			
Rigor ↔ control			
Method			
Human participants			
Data collection			
Results			
Dissemination			

Activity 2

Now that you have thought about the differences between QI, EBP, and research, let's examine some of the similarities. Decide if the following statements about similarities among QI, EBP, and research are *true* (T) or *false* (F).

1. ________ All use a systematic process.
2. ________ Use systematic reasoning to address a clinical issue.
3. ________ All provide evidence for quality care; QI provides the lowest strength and generalizability, whereas research provides the strongest evidence with the greatest generalizability.
4. ________ Results of all three are disseminated, just on a different range.
5. ________ All are collaborative processes.

Activity 3

Quality improvement follows similar steps to the nursing process. In this exercise you will describe how the QI process steps parallel and differ from the nursing process.

Quality Improvement	Nursing Process
	1. Assessment: collecting, organizing, and analyzing information or data about the patient. Subjective or objective data. Collected by observation, interview, examination. Data are reviewed and interpreted. Develop problem list and prioritize patient's problems.
	2. Nursing diagnosis. Statement that describes an actual or potential problem.
	3. Plan. Devise plan using patient goals and nursing orders to provide care that will meet patient's needs. Set patient goals.
	4. Implement. Carry out the nursing care plan you devised. Reassess the patient. Validate that the care plan is accurate. Implement nursing orders. Document.
	5. Evaluate. Compare patient's current status with stated goals. Were goals achieved? Review nursing process.

Activity 4

1. Identify themes for improvement in QI from the following choices. (Select all that apply.)
   a. Eliminating waste
   b. Improving workflow
   c. Optimizing inventory
   d. Changing work environments

e. Production of verifiable knowledge
f. Time management
g. Managing variation
h. Designing systems to avoid mistakes
i. Focusing on products or services

2. Which of the following are external incentives to quality improvement? (Select all that apply.)
   a. Payment
   b. Accreditation
   c. Performance measures
   d. Chart audits

3. Which of the following is an essential signal that performance is below an agreed-on standard?
   a. Quality improvement
   b. Accreditation
   c. Holistic model of improvement
   d. Benchmarking

4. Identify major approaches to manage health care quality. (Select all that apply.)
   a. Total Quality Management/Continuous Quality Improvement
   b. Lean
   c. Six Sigma
   d. Clinical Microsystems model
   e. All of the above
   d. None of the above

5. Common cause variation occurs at ____________ and the solution may require working on multiple causes, whereas special cause variation arises from a special situation that causes disruption ____________ what can be accounted for by random variation.
   a. Predictable intervals, beyond
   b. Random, equal to
   c. Random, beyond
   d. A single point, far above

6. Depicts how a process works, detailing the sequence of steps from the beginning to the end of a process.
   a. Run chart
   b. Flow chart
   c. Control chart
   d. Tree diagram

7. Includes information on the average performance level for the system depicted by a center line displaying the system's average performance (the mean value), and the upper and lower limits depicting 1 to 3 standard deviations from average performance level.
   a. Run chart
   b. Flow chart
   c. Control chart
   d. Tree diagram

8. The vertical axis depicts the value of measure of interest and the horizontal axis depicts the value of each measure running over time.
   a. Run chart
   b. Flow chart
   c. Control chart
   d. Tree diagram

POSTTEST

Use the following items to fill in the blanks of questions 1 to 7. Not all items will be used; some items may be used more than once.

a. Accreditation
b. Assess system performance
c. Analyze data to identify problems
d. Benchmarking
e. Common cause variation
f. Develop a plan
g. Efficient
h. Equitable
i. Effective
j. Families
k. Improvement model
l. Plan-do-study-act
m. Patients
n. Patient-centered
o. Quality health care
p. Safe
q. Support staff
r. SQUIRE
s. Special cause variation
t. Timely
u. Test and implement the improvement plan

1. The following are characteristics of quality health care according to the Institute of Medicine (IOM): care that is __________, ______________________, ________________________________, _____________________, __________________, and ________________________.

2. ______________________________ is one method for tracking performance and knowing when performance is below the accepted standard and in need of QI.

3. The steps of the QI process are: ____, ____________________ ____________________________________, ____, and ____________ ____________________________________.

4. A lead QI team should include representatives from the professions involved in patient care, __________________, __________________________, and ________________________.

5. System variation may be due to random causes or ____________________________ or it may be due to ________________________________.

6. Publication and dissemination of the results of QI studies have been difficult because of the limits on generalizability of this type of work; the ____________________________ guidelines were developed to promote publication of QI studies.

7. *PDSA* stands for ________________ and is part of the ____.

Answer Key

CHAPTER 1

Activity 1

1. c
2. d
3. b
4. a
5. g
6. e
7. f
8. h
9. i
10. j
11. q
12. n
13. o
14. k
15. p
16. m
17. l

Activity 2

1. b
2. b
3. a
4. b
5. a
6. a
7. b

Activity 3

1. Preliminary
2. Comprehensive
3. Parts; whole

Activity 4

1. a. Level IV (repeated measures or longitudinal study)
   b. Level IV (cross-sectional study)
   c. Level 1 (systematic review with meta-analysis)
2. Answers will vary

Activity 5

1. b
2. a
3. c

Activity 6

1. Introduction
2. Abstract, Introduction
3. Introduction
4. Introduction
5. Introduction
6. Abstract, Introduction, Methods
7. Abstract, Methods (Sample & Site), Results (Sample)
8. Not stated
9. Methods (Measures)
10. Methods (Measures)
11. Methods (Procedure)
12. Methods (Data Analysis)
13. Results
14. Discussion
15. Conclusions & limitations

POSTTEST

1. a. Concepts: spiritual/religious coping, grief, depression, PTSD, personal growth
   b. Will vary for each student.
   c. Will vary for each student. Possibilities include the following: How was depression/grief/coping/personal growth defined, and do you agree with that concept? Does a higher or lower score in one item on a scale equal grief, depression, or PTSD? How do the patients define coping, grief, depression, PTSD, and personal growth?
2. Both research and evidence-based practice begin with a question.
3. In research, the question is explored with a design appropriate to the question and specific methodology to contribute to new knowledge. In evidence-based practice, the question is used to guide the search for knowledge (research) to address the question.
4. Both qualitative and quantitative research aim to generate new knowledge using designs appropriate to the question being asked.
5. Qualitative research seeks to interpret the meaning of phenomena, whereas quantitative research seeks to test hypotheses using statistical methods to explore phenomena.

CHAPTER 2

Activity 1

1. f
2. b
3. d
4. a
5. c
6. e

Activity 2

1. c
2. d

Activity 3

1. c
2. a
3. b
4. c
5. c
6. c
7. b
8. a
9. b
10. c

Activity 4

1. yes yes yes
2. yes yes yes
3. yes yes no

Activity 5

1. a. Iron
   b. Iron status
   c. DH
2. a. continuous albuterol (usual or high dose)
   b. peak flow
   c. NDH
3. a. dental prophylaxes
   b. glycemic control
   c. DH
4. a. parenting
   b. blood pressure and heart rate
   c. DH

Activity 6

1. IV
2. Both
3. DV
4. Both
5. IV
6. IV
7. DV
8. DV
9. Both
10. IV
11. DV

Activity 7

1. P = children with long bone fractures in ED
   I = intranasal fentanyl
   C = intravenous morphine
   O = pain control
2. P = obese school-age children and their parents
   I = group intervention
   C = routine care
   O = weight loss
3. P = men after laparoscopic radical prostatectomy
   I = none
   C = none
   O = experiences

POSTTEST

1. F
2. T
3. F
4. T
5. F
6. F
7. T
8. T

CHAPTER 3

Activity 1

1. P
2. P
3. S
4. P

Activity 2

1. B
2. B
3. A
4. B
5. A
6. A

Activity 3

1. C
2. A
3. B

Activity 4

1. C
2. G
3. A
4. I
5. K
6. D
7. L
8. J
9. H
10. E
11. F
12. B

POSTTEST

1. b
2. 1. a
   2. a
   3. a
   4. c
   5. b
3. 1. a
   2. b
   3. a
   4. b
   5. b

4. a
5. c
6. P. Homeless men on parole
   I. Differing levels of peer-coaching and nurse-delivered interventions
   C. Usual care
   O. Completion of the HAV and HBV vaccine series
7. a
8. b

CHAPTER 4

Activity 1

B, C, A

Activity 2

1. e
2. f
3. a
4. b
5. d
6. c
7. g

Activity 3

1. C, B, A
2. C
3. A
4. B
5. C

Activity 4

1. T
2. F
3. T
4. F
5. F
6. F
7. T

Activity 5

a. 3
b. 1
c. 4
d. 2

POSTTEST

1. b, c
2. a
3. c
4. b
5. a
6. a
7. b
8. b
9. f
10. t
11. t
12. f
13. f
14. f
15. t

CHAPTER 5

Activity 1

1. G
2. A
3. C
4. E
5. B
6. H
7. F
8. D
9. J
10. I

Activity 2

	Qualitative	Quantitative
Sample Recruitment	b. Until data saturation	d. Predetermined number of participants
Data Collection	c. Naturalistic setting; numbers	a. Statistics and numbers

Activity 3

Element	Summary
Purpose	The aim of this qualitative study was to explore how patients assign a number on the basis of the NRS (Numeric Rating Scale) to their currently experienced postoperative pain and which considerations influenced this process.
Method	Qualitative research, grounded theory
Sample and Setting	Patients who had surgery the day prior and were currently reporting a NRS score of at least 4. The researcher selected patients purposively to get a diverse sample by sex, age, ethnicity, previous pain experiences, and previous NRS experience. The setting was in a university hospital.
Data Collection	Individual interviews, semi-structured, in-depth. Used open-ended questions.

POSTTEST

1. a. Quantitative
   b. Qualitative
   c. Qualitative
   d. Qualitative
   e. Quantitative
   f. Qualitative

2. (1) Review of the literature: extensive, systematic, critical review of most important published scholarly literature on the topic
   (2) Study design: blueprint for a study
   (3) Sample: representative units from a population, description of process for selection
   (4) Study setting: description of where subjects were recruited and where data collection occurred
   (5) Data collection: description of how informed consent was obtained, what occurred between contact with the participant and the end of the interview, how were data collected, was a recording made, how long was the interview
   (6) Data analysis: how did the researcher take the raw data—words—and analyze them to find commonalities and differences; usually you will find an example
   (7) Findings: a presentation of the results, a description of the phenomenon, and the role or theme

CHAPTER 6

Activity 1

1. d
2. a
3. c
4. e
5. b
6. f
7. g

Activity 2

1. Identifying the phenomenon
   1. E
   2. A
   3. C
   4. D
   5. B
2. Structuring the Study
   1. A
   2. C
   3. B
   4. E
   5. D
3. Data Collection
   1. D
   2. E
   3. A
   4. B
   5. C
4. Data Analysis
   1. A
   2. D
   3. E
   4. C
   5. B
5. Description of the Findings
   1. C
   2. E
   3. B
   4. D
   5. A

Activity 3

1. C
2. B
3. A
4. A
5. B
6. D
7. C
8. A
9. C
10. D
11. C
12. C
13. B
14. A
15. D
16. A (could also be true of B or C)
17. A (could also be true of B or C)
18. C
19. C (could also be true of A)
20. B
21. B

Activity 4

1. b
2. d
3. a
4. a, b, c

POSTTEST

1. T
2. T
3. F
4. T
5. F
6. a
7. d
8. b
9. a
10. c
11. d
12. a, b, d, or f
13. c

CHAPTER 7

Activity 1

1. g
2. e
3. c
4. f
5. d
6. b
7. h
8. f

9. a
10. g
11. h
12. e

Activity 2

1. T
2. T
3. T
4. T

Activity 3

1. B
2. A
3. B
4. C
5. C
6. A
7. C
8. C

POSTTEST

1. t
2. f
3. t
4. f
5. f
6. b
7. a
8. c
9. d

CHAPTER 8

Activity 1

1. h
2. l
3. e
4. k
5. d
6. j
7. b
8. a
9. c
10. f
11. g
12. i

Activity 2

All of the following are threats to internal validity. Threats to internal validity are alternate explanations of the relationship between the variables and they are potential sources of bias.

1. f, h
2. b, l
3. a, j
4. e, i
5. d, k
6. c, g

Activity 3

1. b
2. a
3. b
4. e
5. f
6. c
7. c
8. g
9. f
10. d

Activity 4

Your critique may differ from the critique below. Look for similarities in the major points and refer to your textbook if you have questions.

1. Yes, the design is appropriate. The study authors wanted to evaluate the effectiveness of three levels of peer coaching and nurse-delivered interventions versus usual care on the completion of hepatitis A and B vaccine series and they used a randomized controlled trial to do this.
2. Yes, the methods used for control are consistent with the research design. Control is managed by ruling out extraneous or mediating variables that would compete with the independent variables as an explanation for the study's outcome. Nyamathi et al. maintain control of extraneous variables by using research team training, a dedicated nurse for case management, nurse and peer coach interventionist training, a nurse education session in the peer coaching group, and a health promotion session by a peer councilor in the usual care group, a 20-minute session by a peer councelor and recovery and rehabilitation resources in the usual care group, consistent data collection procedures, and randomization of the sample into groups by urn randomization by age, level of custody, HBV vaccine eligibility, and level of substance abuse.
3. Time, the study collected data at baseline, again at 6 months, and again at 12 months: data collection occurred over a long period. Subject availability: the study used recently paroled, homeless men. Equipment required included questionnaires, telephones, written materials, serum collection materials, and immunization materials.
4. Yes, the problem ties in nicely with the study framework (the Comprehensive Health Seeking and Coping Program). The authors provide a solid literature review as a strong basis for the intervention.
5. Threats to internal validity include: testing, mortality, and selection bias. To reduce the effects of selection bias, participants were randomly assigned to treatment groups. Selection bias was also minimized by clear inclusion and exclusion criteria. To reduce the effects of mortality, the research team created a locator guide to help find participants who moved or were no longer in the program office near the study office. Testing may have influenced the results in the self-report measures.

6. Selection, reactive effects, measurement effects
   a. Selection: sample was comprised of homeless men on parole in a single county.
   b. Reactive effects: it is possible that there could have been some positive outcomes simply from being included in the study and receiving health promotion sessions.
   c. Measurement: the participants knew that they were being monitored; however, vaccine series completion was monitored by a vaccine tracking system not self-report.

Activity 5

1. T. Since your population of interest was not included in the study, you would not include the data from this study in the evidence reviewed for your problem. However, the literature cited by the author in the literature review may be a source of information for your review and should be investigated further.
2. T. You would probably choose to trust that intervention fidelity was maintained if you felt that the steps taken, and described, in the report were adequate.
3. F. A negative finding in your area is just as important as a positive finding. Your critiquing criteria would assess validity of the study, any potential weaknesses would be noted, and the results would be included in your evidence.
4. F. You would likely need help from a librarian to develop a literature search to identify populations similar to your population. You would decide if the included studies were clinically relevant to your population.

POSTTEST

1. a. Control
   b. Constancy
   c. External validity
   d. Maturation
   e. Feasibility
   f. Internal validity
   g. Selection bias

CHAPTER 9

Activity 1

1. Experimental
2. Solomon four-group
3. Time series
4. After-only
5. After-only nonequivalent control group
6. True experimental
7. Nonequivalent control group

Activity 2

1. a. Yes.
   b. All of the elements were used in the study.
2. a
3. e
4. Independent variables (IV) include: intensive peer coaching and nurse case management, intensive peer coaching with minimal nurse-delivered interventions, and usual care. Dependent variables (DV) include: completion of the HAV and HBV vaccine series

Activity 3

1.

	Pretest	Teaching	Posttest
Group A	X	X	X
Group B		X	X
Group C	X		X
Group D			X

Note: The groups may be arranged in any order, but the four-group pattern must be followed.

2. a, c
3. b
4. e
5. b
6. d
7. f
8. a

Activity 4

1. All of the items should be marked
2. a
3. d

Activity 5: Evidence-Based Practice Activity

1. Level V
2. Level I
3. Level VI
4. Level II
5. Level III

POSTTEST

1. a. E
   b. Q
   c. E
   d. E
   e. Q
2. a. 3
   b. 1
   c. 2
   d. 6
   e. 4
   f. 5

CHAPTER 10

Activity 1

1. f
2. e
3. c

4. d
5. b
6. c
7. e
8. f
9. b
10. a

Activity 2

	Advantages	Disadvantages
Correlation studies	A3	D1, D3, D4, D7
Cross-sectional	A1, A8	D2, D5
Ex post facto	A4	D1, D2, D3, D4, D5, D7
Longitudinal	A2, A6	D2, D8, D9
Prospective	A2, A7	D3, D4, D7, D8
Retrospective	A4	D1, D2, D3, D4, D5, D7
Survey	A1	D5, D7

Activity 3

1. ES: Exploratory survey
2. L: Longitudinal, or P: prospective
3. CS: Cross-sectional
4. R: Retrospective, or E: Ex post facto
5. C: Correlational
6. M: Methodological
7. MA: Meta-analysis

Activity 4

1. e
2. No
3. Inclusion criteria: English speaking Canadian families with an adolescent (13-20 years old) who completed treatment for a solid tumor, leukemia, or lymphoma 2-10 years earlier at a children's hospital.
   Exclusion criteria: Cancer relapse, organ transplantation, a brain tumor that required only surgery, or significant cognitive or neurologic impairments.
   The inclusion criteria were chosen to try to find PTG that has been theorized to occur after a long process of crisis resolution and recovery.
   The exclusion criteria were chosen because they could represent another crisis or traumatic event. The aims of the study would be harder to demonstrate if the exclusion criteria were not used and they confounded the data.
4. Data were collected from the participants at one point during weeks 24-28 of their pregnancy. Additional data were collected from the medical record during this period and also within 48 hours of delivery.

Activity 5

Ex post facto design

Activity 6: Evidence-Based Practice Activity

1. d
2. b
3. a, b

POSTTEST

1. Variables
2. Survey
3. Descriptive, exploratory, comparative
4. Relationship-difference
5. Correlational
6. Interrelational
7. Retrospective
8. a. Cross-sectional
   b. Longitudinal/prospective
   c. Retrospective/ex post facto
9. Cross-sectional; longitudinal
10. Prospective
11. Retrospective
12. Methodological

CHAPTER 11

Activity 1

1. Meta-analysis, systematic review
2. Integrative review
3. Meta-analysis
4. Clinical practice guidelines
5. Expert-based guidelines, evidence-based guidelines

Activity 2

1. c
2. a
3. e
4. b
5. d

Activity 3

1. SR, MA, IR
2. SR, IR
3. MA
4. IR
5. ECG, EBCG
6. EBCG
7. MA
8. ECG
9. ECG, EBCG
10. IR
11. MA

Activity 4

1. Systematic reviews can provide evidence for developing practice; reviews based on multiple RCTs provide stronger evidence. A meta-analysis can provide Level I evidence, the higher level of evidence. Systematic reviews can help clinicians to manage the expanding volume of research literature. The systematic review process and critiquing process help clinicians

understand how to rate and use the information gleaned from multiple studies.
2. Clinical expertise and patient values or preference
3. b and d
4.

Level of Evidence	Description	Source
Level I	Meta-analysis of RCTs	C
Level II	A well-designed RCT	C
Level III	Quasi-experimental study	C
Level IV	Single nonexperimental study	C
Level V	Systematic review of qualitative studies	B, C
Level VI	Single descriptive or qualitative study	A
Level VII	Opinion of authorities, report of expert committee	A, E

POSTTEST

1. Integrative review
2. Quantitative
3. Systematic review and meta-analysis, meta-analysis
4. More than 1 person, excluded
5. Meta-analysis, highest level of evidence
6. Analysis
7. Bias
8. Forest plot, blobbogram
9. Evidence-based practice, expert-based guidelines
10. Does not, published studies

CHAPTER 12

Activity 1

1. Sample: Set of units that are selected to represent an entire population.
   Population: Well-defined set that has certain specified properties, may be defined broadly or narrowly.
   Differences: The population is the entire set of units with specified characteristics. The entire population is not often feasible to include in a study. The sample is a subset of the population that is selected to represent the entire population.
2. Target population: The entire population that meets the sampling criteria.
   Accessible population: A population that meets the target population criteria and that is available to the researcher.
   Differences: The target population is the whole, whereas the accessible population is the slice that is available to the researcher.
3. Inclusion criteria: Population descriptors used to select a sample.
   Exclusion criteria: Characteristics that restrict the population to make it more homogeneous.
   Differences: These terms describe the same concept. Inclusion, exclusion, eligibility, and delimitations are all terms used to describe subject attributes that researchers consider when determining if the individual is part of a population.

Activity 2

1. Probability sampling uses random selection and is more rigorous. Nonprobability sampling uses nonrandom methods and there is no way to ensure that each element has a chance for inclusion in the sample.
2. a. N
   b. N
   c. P
   d. N
   e. P
   f. P

Activity 3

1. b
2. d
3. a
4. c
5. d
6. e
7. d

Activity 4

1. a. Yes, the sample is adequately described. The inclusion criteria were: parents of a deceased newborn from a singleton pregnancy, lived more than 2 hours in the NICU or deceased infant/child was 18 years or younger and a patient in the PICU for at least 2 hours. Parents had to understand English or Spanish. The exclusion criteria were: Multiple gestation pregnancy if the deceased was a newborn, being in a foster home before hospitalization, injuries suspected to be due to child abuse, and death of a parent in the illness/injury event.
   b. Maybe, there were no statistical analyses run to evaluate differences between the 348 families contacted and the 188 families of those who signed consent forms, and the 124 families who completed the surveys.
   c. Convenience
   d. Nonprobability
   e. C
   f. 114 mothers and 51 fathers from 124 families.
2. Subjects were accessible to the researcher, the researcher was able to assemble a sample meeting the inclusion criteria, and was able to get preliminary data on spiritual coping following the death of an infant/child.
3. Greater risk of bias, voluntary participation may skew results, less generalizability than other sampling methods

Activity 5

1. True
2. True

3. False
4. False
5. True
6. True
7. False

Activity 6

1. g
2. a
3. h
4. k
5. b
6. f
7. c
8. j
9. d
10. e
11. i

Activity 7: Evidence-Based Practice Activity

The sample and sampling strategy is one variable that will influence the strength of the evidence provided by the study. The evidence from a meta-analysis of all *randomized* controlled trials is more influential in making practice change decisions than from a single descriptive or qualitative study with a convenience sample.

POSTTEST

1. Power analysis
2. Probability; nonprobability
3. Convenience
4. Simple random
5. Table of random numbers
6. Stratified random
7. Inclusion, exclusion criteria
8. Convenience, quota, purposive
9. Multistage or cluster
10. Data saturation

CHAPTER 13

Activity 1

1. d. Nursing research committee
2. g. Institutional review board
3. b. Justice
4. e. Expedited review
5. h. Unethical research study
6. i. HIPAA

Activity 2

Can be in any order,
1. a. Beneficence
2. b. Justice
3. j. Respect for person

Activity 3

Elements of Informed Consent

1. √ Title of protocol
2. √ Invitation to participate
3. 0 Basis for subject selection
4. √ Overall purpose of the study
5. √ Explanation of benefits
6. √ Description of risks and discomforts
7. √ Potential benefits
8. 0 Alternatives to participation
9. √ Financial obligations
10. √ Assurance of confidentiality
11. 0 In case of injury compensation
12. 0 HIPAA disclosure
13. √ Subject withdrawal
14. √ Offer to answer questions
15. √ Concluding consent statement
16. √ Identification of investigators

Activity 4

Correct responses include: the elderly, children, pregnant women, the unborn, those who are emotionally or physically disabled, prisoners, the deceased, students, and people with AIDS; also potentially includes oversubscribed research populations (organ transplantation patients, AIDS patients, "captive" and convenient populations).

Activity 5

1. a, c, d, f, g
2. a, b, c, d, f, g (Also, presume "e" was not adhered to because the study began in 1932 before IRBs and formal consent were required.)

Activity 6

1. Appendix A, Nyamathi et al., in the "Design" section under "Methods," write, "The study was approved by the University of California, Los Angeles Institutional Review Board and registered with Clinical Trials. gov (NCT01844414). "Under "Sample and Site,'" write, "Among interested participants, an informed consent was signed that allowed the research staff to administer a brief screening questionnaire to assess eligibility criteria. Among participants who met eligibility criteria, a second informed consent allowed administration of a baseline questionnaire; a detailed locator guide allows participants to fill out contact information, addresses, and phone numbers for research staff to follow-up."
2. Appendix B, Hawthorne et al., document in the "Procedure" section of the article that "The study was approved by the Institutional Review Boards (IRB) from the University, the 4 recruitment facilities, and the State Department of Health prior to recruitment of study participants. A clinical co-investigator from each NICU/PICU identified eligible families. The project director sent a letter to each family (Spanish on one side and English on the other) describing the study and called the family to explain the study. Of the 348 families contacted for the larger study, 188 (54%) families signed consent forms for their participation and review of their deceased child's medical record. The SCS was added to the study after 64 families

were recruited. The remaining 124 families completed the SCS."
3. Appendix C, van Dijk et al., report in the "Methods" section under "Participants," "All 27 patients who were asked agreed to participate, and written informed consent was obtained. The study was approved by the medical ethics committee of the University Medical Centre Utrecht in which the study took place."
4. Appendix D, Turner-Sack et al., state in the "Methods" section under "Procedure" that "Following institutional ethics approvals from the University of Windsor in Ontario, Canada and the University of Western Ontario in London, Ontario, Canada, data were collected from the pediatric oncology population at Children's Hospital of Western Ontario in London, Ontario, Canada. Questionnaires were mailed to 89 families that met criteria for the study. They were informed that participants' names would be entered into a drawing for a $50 gift certificate from a local store."

Activity 7: Evidence-Based Practice Activity

You could check the *Federal Register* or other government documents or websites to determine if misconduct had occurred, or check the journal for a correction or follow-up research report.

POSTTEST

1. Yes, because extra precautions should be taken to protect the rights of vulnerable populations, but this would not preclude undertaking research.
2. Before
3. Informed consent documents, IRB approval from the appropriate agency.
4. Yes
5. Informed consent
6. Risks to subjects may be greater than benefits, a patient's basic human rights could be violated, and results of a study would be questionable.

CHAPTER 14

Activity 1

Study 1 (Thomas et al.)

1. e, d
2. Vaccine completion was assessed by a vaccine tracking system; the advantage of using this system is that it removes the chance of misreporting due to social desirability. Instruments used to collect data also included a structured questionnaire to collect sociodemographic information, a baseline questionnaire assessed homeless status, history of criminal activity, and severity of criminal history, contract type, and time in RDT. Other instruments included Texas Christian University Drug History form, General health 5 point scale, Hostility subscale of the Brief Symptom Inventory, Center for Epidemiological Studies Depression Scale short-form, Medical Outcomes Study Social Support Survey, and the Carver Brief Cope Instrument. Questionnaires are particularly useful for collecting data on experiences, feelings, behaviors, or attitudes. The researchers were looking at predictors of vaccine completion and wanted measures of situational factors, personal factors, and social factors but they also needed to be cognizant of participant time so many short forms or single item scales were utilized. The researchers were aware of the difficulty in keeping contact with this population, thus to keep in touch, they had participants fill out a locator guide so that future assessments could continue, part of keeping contact was having the nurse or peer coach send reminders about the next dose and appointment cards.

Study 2 (Hawthrone et al.)

1. d, e
2. The researchers wanted to understand the relationships between spiritual/religious coping strategies and grief, mental health, and personal growth for mothers and fathers over time after the death of a child. Data were collected from the child's medical record and also by questionnaires administered by the researcher in the family's home or another place of their choosing. Instruments included the Hogan Grief Reaction Checklist, Beck Depression Inventory, Impact of Events Scale-Revised, and the Spiritual Coping Strategies scale. Mental health, spiritual/religious coping, and personal growth are an experience, feeling, behavior, or attitude and a questionnaire is the appropriate method for collecting these data. The medical record contains the record of infant/child gender, age, and cause of death and is the appropriate place to collect this type of data.

Study 3 (van Dijk et al.)

1. c, d
2. The researchers wanted to understand how patients assign a number to the currently experienced postoperative pain. Interviews were conducted using semi-structured, in-depth interviews on the day after surgery. Questions were open ended. Interviewers used a topic guide developed based on the literature, nursing experts, and preliminary studies. Interviews were recorded and transcribed verbatim. The researchers also used a structured questionnaire to collect age, gender, ethnicity, surgical procedure, chronic pain, and education. The interview method provides the most flexibility when used with open-ended questions to learn about the experience of assigning a number for pain. One weakness of using a small sample such as this is that it lacks generalizability and may not be representative of the experience of all patients who experience postoperative pain.

Study 4 (Turner-Sack et al.)

1. d
2. The surveys used included: a background questionnaire (age, gender, ethnicity, education, type of cancer, age at diagnosis, time since diagnosis, time since treatment

completion, and type of treatment), the Brief Symptom Inventory, Student's Life Satisfaction Scale, Satisfaction with Life Scale, Post Traumatic Growth Inventory, and the COPE.

3. Possible answers: the sample relied on self report and the sample was skewed to a primarily middle-class, European/Canadian population. Also, the researchers did not obtain surveys only from parent/child dyads and the results reflect many different families and primarily mothers not fathers, so they may not have captured a family-systems perspective.

Activity 2

1. b. Consumers
2. l. Physiological
3. m. Reactivity
4. f. Interviews
5. n. Records
6. j. Questionnaire
7. h. Objectivity, d. consistency
8. c. Concealment
9. k. Participant observation
10. i. Operationalization
11. g. Likert scale
12. e. Content analysis

Activity 3

1. Children; interactions between people where the investigator is not part of the interaction; psychiatric patients; classrooms
2. The consent is usually of the type where permission to observe for a specified purpose is requested. The specific behaviors that are to be observed are not named. The use of the data and degree of anonymity are explained. In some situations, the subjects will be asked to review the data after the observation and before inclusion in the data pool.
3. Reactivity is the major concern, when the investigator has reason to believe that his or her presence will change the nature of the subjects' behavior.

Activity 4

1. d
2. a
3. d
4. a, b, c
5. d

Activity 5: Evidence-Based Practice Activity

Answers will vary depending on the topic chosen, when the search is conducted, and what database is used.

POSTTEST

1. d
2. d
3. c
4. b
5. b
6. d
7. c
8. d
9. b
10. b
11. b
12. d
13. a
14. d
15. a

CHAPTER 15

Activity 1

1. S; avoided by proper calibration of the scale.
2. S; decrease error by providing instructions, ensuring confidentiality, or other means to allow students to freely express themselves.
3. R; lessen by training research assistants and using strict protocols or rulebooks to guide analysis.
4. R; decrease their anxiety by addressing their concerns, providing comfort measures, or other efforts that might decrease their anxiety. Anxiety may alter the test responses.

Activity 2

1. a. Construct validity
2. g. Face validity
3. a. Content validity
4. b. Content validity index
5. a. Construct validity or d. convergent validity
6. d. Convergent validity; c. contrasted groups; f. divergent validity; h. factor analysis; i. hypothesis testing
7. c. Contrasted groups

Activity 3

1. g, d, c
2. h. Test-retest methods could be accomplished by giving the same test again at a later date and seeing if the two scores are highly correlated.
   f. Parallel or alternate forms, such as alternate versions of the same test, could also be used to establish stability.
3. Alternate forms would be better if the test-taker is likely to remember and be influenced by the items or the answers from the first test.
4. a. 2
   b. 4
   c. 1
   d. 3
5. a. (2) A Likert scale is commonly used when measuring psychosocial variables or attitudes. It asks respondents to respond to a question using a scale of varying intensity between two extremes. We would expect the scale to ask if the respondent strongly agrees or disagrees with a statement or if the statement is "most like me or least like me" on a scale from 1-5 where 1 is anchored by being least like me.

b. (5) Cronbach's alpha. This is the most commonly used measure for Likert type scales.
c. (6) Reliability. Measures of internal consistency help provide the reader with an idea of the reliability of the measures used.
d. (9) Alphas above .70 are sufficient evidence for supporting the internal consistency of the instrument.

Activity 4

1. Four instruments, Hogan Grief Reaction Checklist (HGRC), Beck Depression Inventory (BDI-II), Impact of Events Scale–Revised (IES-R), Spiritual Coping Strategies Scale (SCS), and a demographic questionnaire developed for this study.
2. a. (1) No specific information on validity was given.
   b. (3) Cronbach's alpha
   c. (3) Cronbach's alpha, (4) test-retest reliability, (5) item-total correlations and (6) inter-item correlations for each domain in the scale, (7) split-half, parallel or (8) alternate form.
   d. (1) No, it is used for yes/no format questionnaires; the BDI-II uses a 3-point Likert scale.
   e. (1) No, at least not reported as such by the authors
   f. You would start with the reference given for reliability and validity and you may complete a search of reliability and validity on this instrument.
   g. You would read the discussion section; the authors do compare their results to other studies and discuss the differences on subscale scores. This is also a good place to look for discussion about threats to internal or external validity.

Activity 5: Evidence-Based Practice Activity

First, this study would need to be put into context. It would need to be known what other studies were available in the same area. If a decision were being made based solely on the published reliability and validity information, it would not be considered a strong study.

To qualify this statement, there may be more information about the reliability and validity of the instruments. Some of it may have been cut to meet required article length. Some information is given, and what is presented is valuable and does lead to some confidence in the results—certainly more confidence than if they had been using several newly constructed instruments.

A final answer would be "it depends." Some questions would need to be asked and a deeper literature search on adolescent cancer survivors and their families would need to be done.

POSTTEST

1. f. Cronbach's alpha
2. i. Concurrent
3. c. Convergent
4. a. Content
5. b. Factor analysis
6. h. Interrater
7. e. Test-retest
8. a. Content
9. c. Convergent
10. f. Cronbach's alpha

CHAPTER 16

Activity 1

1. d
2. c
3. d
4. a
5. a, b, or c, depending on the tool used to measure satisfaction
6. a
7. b
8. d
9. a
10. c
11. d

Activity 2

1. c
2. b
3. e
4. i
5. a
6. d
7. h
8. j
9. f
10. c
11. c
12. g

Activity 3

1. a. Psychological functioning, posttraumatic growth, coping, and cancer-related characteristics
   b. Treated as an interval level variable
2. a. Spiritual coping
   b. Grief, mental health, and personal growth
   c. In order to use inferential statistics, we know that it must be at interval or ratio level. The SCS used a Likert scale and there is no stated absolute zero, so it must be interval level.
3. a. A dyad is two individuals who are regarded as a pair in the analysis. The authors want to understand the family dynamic of parents, siblings, and cancer survivors.
   b. This is a test of the difference between groups.

Activity 4

1. d. Null hypothesis
2. f. Parametric statistics
3. i. Research hypothesis
4. j. Sampling error
5. e. *Parameter*; k. *statistic*
6. b. Correlation
7. n. Type II error; m. type I error

8. h. Probability
9. g. Practical significance
10. c. Nonparametric statistics
11. l. Statistical significance
12. i. Research hypothesis; d. null hypothesis

Activity 5

1. a. Yes
   b. Yes
   c. Yes
   d. Yes
2. All studies used descriptive statistics to describe certain characteristics of the sample (e.g., age, sex, ethnicity, marital status, income).
   a. Social characteristics, situational characteristics, coping, personal characteristics, sample size (N), mean, standard deviation (SD), range
   b. Education, partnered, employed, religion, N, mean, SD, range, median
   c. Age at diagnosis, time since diagnosis, treatment duration, education, diagnosis, treatment, N, frequency, %
   d. Surgical type, chronic pain, N, %, mean, SD, Z score
3. a. Yes
   b. Yes
   c. Yes
   d. Yes
4. Yes, the Hawthorne et al. and Turner-Sack et al. studies were descriptive studies.
5. a. Yes
   b. Yes
   c. No
   d. Yes
6. a. Chi square (χ^2), ANOVA, two-sample tests, multiple logistic regression analysis, Hosmer-Lemeshow test
   b. Pearson correlation, multiple regression analyses
   c. None used because this is a qualitative study
   d. Pearson product moment correlation, standard regression with forward entry, independent sample *t* tests

Optional Flash Card Activity 6

You will have a set of reference cards that can also serve as flashcards.

POSTTEST

1. This is a matter of personal preference and of probability. At clinic 1 you would have a longer average wait time, but 68% of the wait times would be from 30 to 50 minutes. At clinic 2, you may have a shorter wait sometimes, but 68% of the wait times would be between 0 and 70 minutes.
2. The mean would provide information about the most common number of hospital gowns needed on your unit, but it is sensitive to outliers. The median could also be examined, but it is not clear if the hospital gown data have a normal distribution. Perhaps the best method would be to look at both the mean and median to determine the number of gowns for your unit. The mode may be useful, but again without knowing the distribution of the data, there is no way to know if the gown data have one mode or are bimodal. The mode would be less useful than the median and mean.
3. Mode------------------Most frequent score
   Median----------------Middle score
   Mean-------------------Arithmetical average – most stable
4. e. Nonsymmetrical, g. positive, d. negative
5. b. Hypothesis
6. h. Sampling distributions, c. inferential
7. f. Null hypothesis
8. i. Type II error
9. a. χ^2
10. c, b, a, e, d

CHAPTER 17

Activity 1

1. R
2. D
3. R
4. D
5. R
6. R
7. D

Activity 2

1. d
2. b
3. a
4. e
5. c

Activity 3

1. T
2. F
3. F
4. T
5. T
6. F

POSTTEST

1. b
2. a
3. c, d
4. a, a, a
5. b
6. a
7. a
8. a

CHAPTER 18

Activity 2

Please note that what follows are the results of one inspectional reading of the study by Nyamathi et al. (2015). You are not expected to agree with these findings. Some of you may agree, but some of you may not.

Systematic skimming: In reading the title, abstract, the biographies, and the discussion, the following conclusions were made:

The biographical information of the authors/researchers indicates that they have a clinical nursing background in substance abuse, sociology, and research/statistical methods.

The PICO of the scenario could be P: homeless clients at risk for hepatitis infection, I: nurse-led interventions, C: usual care, O: hepatitis vaccine series completion. The PICO of the study is similar to the PICO from the scenario. The PICO from the study would be P: homeless men on parole; I_1: peer coaching, I_2: nurse case management + peer coaching; C: hepatitis vaccine series completion and predictors of completion.

Yes, would proceed to superficial reading.

Superficial reading:

1. Remembered about the study:
   - Two interventions, one control group; an experimental study
   - Hypotheses
   - 345 male parolees randomly assigned to one of three groups
   - There was randomization
   - Reliable and valid data collection tools, references provided
   - This would be level II evidence
   - The study was approved by an ethics board
   - Figures and tables with data
   - Data analysis section
   - Results section
   - Discussion section
   - Reread this study in greater detail and consider for critical appraisal. It continues to appear to be relevant to the scenario.

Activity 3

An experimental study of moderate to strong quality, given that the strengths outweigh the limitations, was conducted in a sample of homeless men on parole who were seronegative for hepatitis. Participants were randomly assigned to receive one of two interventions (peer coaching or peer coaching plus nurse case management) or usual care. There were no significant differences between the groups for vaccine completion, and completion rates were 73% for all groups. Predictors of vaccine completion were having six or more friends, recent cocaine use, and staying in drug treatment at least 90 days, whereas vaccine noncompletion was associated with being Asian and Pacific Islander, experiencing high levels of hostility, social support, injection drug use, early prison release, and admission for psychiatric illness. Based on the findings of this one study, a recommendation is made to focus on screening individuals for high risk for vaccine noncompletion.

CHAPTER 19

Activity 1

1. a. P—older adults
   b. I—frequency and duration of social interaction
   c. C—none*
   d. O—mortality
   e. Prognosis
2. a. P—patients with diabetic foot ulcers without arterial insufficiency
   b. I—hyperbaric oxygen treatment
   c. C—wound coverage by cultured cells
   d. O—wound healing
   e. Therapy
3. a. P—adolescent clinical patients
   b. I—self report measures
   c. C—none*
   d. O—screening for substance abuse
   e. Diagnosis
4. a. P—children
   b. I—residential exposure to low level radio frequency radiation from smart meters
   c. C—none*
   d. O—brain or cental nervous system cancers
   e. Causation/Harm

*Note in some studies, there is no comparison.

Activity 2

1. Therapy; Prognosis; Causation; Review; Qualitative
2. Clinical Trial; Meta-Analysis; Practice Guideline; Randomized Controlled Trial
3. Etiology; Diagnosis; Therapy; Prognosis; Clinical Predication Guides
4. PUBMED (Medline) —"Clinical Queries"

Activity 3

1. g
2. c
3. h
4. a
5. e
6. j
7. b
8. f
9. i
10. k
11. d

Activity 4

1. The percentage of patients who reported 7-day tobacco abstinence 9 months after randomization; (b) discrete/dichotomous.
2. 1.0. Note: The null value varies depending on the outcome; for a continuous outcome variable, the null value would be 0.0.
3. We are 95% certain that when a patient receives the smoking cessation intervention they will be anywhere from 1.5 to 4 times more likely to stop smoking than patients who did not receive the intervention.

4. Patients receiving care from the smoking cessation intervention team are 2.5 times mre likely to quit than patients receiving usual care. The OR (or treatment effect) is statistically significant because the 95% CI (1.5, 4.0) does not include 1.0 (the null value).
5. Ten patients need to be treated with the smoking cessation program in order to stop 1 patient from smoking. The NNT was calculated first by finding the absolute risk reduction (ARR), then dividing 1 by the ARR. A lower NNT means that less patients will need to be treated to get one patient to stop smoking. In this study, we would look at the cost of the intervention and the human resources needed to deliver the intervention to determine if 1 patient giving up smoking for every 10 who receive the intervention is beneficial enough to justify the cost.
6. Although there was a significant reduction in smoking among patients who received the, intervention program there is likely research evidence to support alternate tobacco cessation strategies in the given scenario. However, in continuing the implementation, the RN should consider if (a) the population in the study is similar to his or her clinical situation (target population) and that (b) the application of results of the study to the target population should be done with caution until higher level evidence (i.e., systematic review, practice guideline) is available.

Activity 5

1. P—pediatric patients; I—parental consumption of artificially sweetened beverages; C—no consumption; O—child obesity
2. There would be concern that the difference in ages of the target population (children) and study population (infants) would be significantly different even though the clinical situation PICO question and study question are similar. Also, the PICO question addressed consumption by both parents while the study specifically looked at maternal consumption during pregnancy.
3. Causation because the clinical situation and study are about determining whether one thing is related to another; based on the study design (cohort study) you would select the CASP Tool for Cohort Studies.
4. a. Discrete/dichotomous
   b. continuous
   c. Discrete/dichotomous
5. Daily consumption of artificially sweetened beverages during pregnancy was associated with 2 times higher risk for your infant to be overweight at 1 year of age; the null value is 1.0; the CI for the variable of infant BMI z score do not include 1.0, indicating that these results are statistically significant.
6. Although results of this study reflect a population of infants in Canada, it is possible that there may be credibility in applying the evidence to the current clinical situation. Although an evidence-based practice change may not be warranted by this one study, a further review, critical appraisal, and synthesis of the evidence could lead to changes in counseling parents about artificially sweetened beverages and childhood obesity in the target population.

POSTTEST

1. False; an experimental or quasiexperimental study design is usually used for the therapy category of clinical concern used by clinicians; causation/harm studies typically use nonexperimental (longitudinal or retrospective) study designs.
2. True
3. True
4. False; sensitivity is the proportion of those with the disease who test positive, and specificity is the proportion of those without the disease who test negative.
5. False; the CI provides the reader information about both the statistical and clinical significance of the findings. Although findings may be statistically significant, the clinician must apply the "low" and "high" end of the confidence levels to determine clinical significance.
6. True
7. True
8. False; *likelihood ratio* is a term used to describe the number that expresses the sensitivity, specificity, PPV, NPV, and prevalence for diagnosis clinical category questions.

CHAPTER 20

Activity 1

1. 1. a
   2. b
   3. b
   4. a
   5. a
2. a. The best available evidence
   b. Clinical expertise
   c. Patient values

Activity 2

1. b
2. d
3. a
4. c
5. b
6. d

Activity 3

a. 4
b. 1
c. 5
d. 10
e. 2

f. 11
g. 7
h. 9
i. 3
j. 6
k. 8

Activity 4

1. b, e
2. c
3. a, d, g, f

Activity 5

1. Y
2. N
3. Y
4. N
5. N
6. Y

Activity 6

1. a. The nature of the innovation (e.g., the type and strength of evidence)
   b. The manner in which the innovation is communicated
2. a. 3
   b. 4
   c. 1
   d. 2
3. a. Y
   b. Y
   c. N
   d. Y

POSTTEST

1. This was a test of implementation of an evidence-based program, FOCUS, for cancer survivors and their caregivers in a small group format.
2. All clinicians at the agency offering the program are master's-level social workers. Modifications were made to the FOCUS program through collaboration with the research staff who developed the program. The program director shadowed a FOCUS intervention nurse conducting a separate study to observe interactions and understand the program. The research team from FOCUS met with the program director weekly to discuss modifications to the FOCUS program.
3. It appears that all members of the team could be considered stakeholders; key stakeholders not represented could include patients, patient caregivers, patients' families, senior hospital leadership (both medical and nursing), and nearby health systems with patients who may be eligible for referral to this program.
4. Not indicated, most likely because this study was focused on implementation, not the evidence-based practice (EBP) problem.
5. Not indicated, most likely because this study was focused on implementation, not the EBP problem.
6. Not indicated, most likely because this study was focused on implementation, not the EBP problem.
7. Not indicated, most likely because this study was focused on implementation, not the EBP problem.
8. To a degree; however, recommendations are missing an indication to the evidence to support the recommendations and the grade of the evidence.
9. Somewhat; the authors point to the available research on the efficacy of the FOCUS program and they note the lack of evidence on the effectiveness of the program.
10. Detailed methodology for determining feasibility includes measurements of enrollment and retention rates, intervention fidelity, and participant satisfaction with the program.
11. Yes; yes, the authors report several positive outcomes.
    "Feasibility was examined by enrollment and retention rates, intervention fidelity, and satisfaction. The enrollment rate was 60%, and retention rate was 92%. Intervention fidelity was assessed by the number of interventions listed in the FOCUS Protocol Checklist that were checked as completed in each intervention group by the social worker who led the group. A total of 77 interventions are listed in the protocol checklist, and 73 interventions (on average across intervention groups) were marked as completed, indicating high intervention fidelity of 94%. Both survivors and caregivers reported high satisfaction with the program on the 5-item satisfaction scale. Survivors' and caregivers' mean satisfaction scores did not differ significantly (survivors: 4.26 [SD, 0.8]; caregivers: 4. 34 [SD, 0.7]). In addition, the majority of survivors (88.2%) and caregivers (85.7%) said the program helped them to cope with the cancer, and most survivors (88.6%) and caregivers (82.9%) also said the program did not duplicate anything they received from their cancer center. Nearly all survivors and caregivers (97.1% each) said that they would recommend the program to other cancer survivors and their family caregivers."
12. CSC director could be considered both "Change Champion" (as a result of clinical expertise qualities) and "Opinion Leader" (because of technological qualities), both of which encompass EBP expertise; didactic education (education during the FOCUS training program).

CHAPTER 21

Activity 1

Your answers may vary.

	Quality Improvement	Evidence-Based Practice	Research
Purpose	Improve internal practices or processes	Change or reinforce nursing practice	Generate knowledge
Rigor ↔ Control	Protocols less formal/rigorous, may change throughout project	Interventions are more strict than QI, but not as controlled as research	Tight control of variables
Method	Total Quality Management/ Continuous Quality Improvement (TQM/CQI) Six Sigma Lean Clinical Microsystems	Iowa model of EBP Johanna Briggs Institute model of EBP	Qualitative, quantitative, or mixed methods
Human participants	Doesn't usually require institutional review board (IRB) approval	Doesn't usually require IRB approval	Requires IRB approval unless exempt
Data collection	Benchmarking Collecting and monitoring data Rapid cycle	Literature search and appraisal Data collection not as rapid as QI	Observation, self-report, physiological, medical records, databases Data collection time varies
Results	Improve process	Treatments or nursing care are based on the best available evidence	Adds to the body of scientific knowledge
Dissemination	Within a unit or an agency	Publications, conferences, consultations, training programs, changing practitioner behavior through interaction with those who provide direct care	Scientific community, publications, conferences

Activity 2

Your answers may vary.

1. T
2. T
3. T
4. T
5. T

Activity 3

You may fit the steps into the table differently, but be sure that all of the QI steps are included.

Quality Improvement	Nursing Process
1. Assess system performance by collecting/monitoring data. Data may include check or data sheets, surveys, interviews, or focus groups.	1. Assessment: collecting, organizing, and analyzing information or data about the patient. Subjective or objective data. Collected by observation, interview, examination. Data are reviewed and interpreted. Develop problem list and prioritize patient's problems.
2. Analyze data to ID problems in need of improvement. Determine if problem is due to common cause or special cause variation. Methods for analysis include run charts, control charts, histograms, pie or bar charts, cause/effect diagrams, fishbone diagrams, RCA, tree diagram, 5 whys, flow chart.	2. Nursing diagnosis. Statement that describes an actual or potential problem.
3. Develop a plan for improvement. Develop and test a plan to treat the performance problem. May use the Model of Improvement.	3. Plan. Devise plan using patient goals and nursing orders to provide care that will meet patient's needs. Set patient goals.
4. Test and implement the plan. Use the PDSA cycle; use small and rapid tests of change. Evaluate success of the intervention, monitor system performance, track stability and sustainability of your change.	4. Implement. Carry out the nursing care plan you devised. Reassess the patient. Validate that the care plan is accurate. Implement nursing orders. Document.
5. Continue test and implement phase. Monitor system performance over time. Compare results to baseline.	5. Evaluate. Compare patient's current status with stated goals. Were goals achieved? Review nursing process.

Activity 4

1. All but e
2. All but d
3. d
4. e
5. c
6. b
7. c
8. a

POSTTEST

1. o, i, n, t, g, h
2. d
3. b, c, f, u
4. q, m, j
5. e, s
6. r
7. l, k